USMLE®* Step 2 CS

STRATEGIES, PRACTICE, & REVIEW

KAPLAN

MEDICAL

Published by Kaplan Medical, a division of Kaplan, Inc.
750 Third Avenue,
New York, NY 10017

Printed in the United States of America
10 9 8 7 6 5 4 3 2 1

Course ISBN: 978-1-62523-906-8 | Item Number: CS5009F

Retail ISBN: 978-1-62523-715-6

EDITORS

Mariana Cuceu, M.D.

Edward Kalpas, M.D.

Phyllis Levine, M.D.

CONTRIBUTORS

Eugene Festa, M.D., Ph.D.

Neelam G. Gidwaney, M.D.

Miguel Rubina, M.D.

Maybeth Ryan

Nambirajan (Raj) Srinivasan, M.D.

Michelle Una'dia, M.D.

Elsa Varghese, M.D.

Sherine Elsayegh, M.D.

CURRICULUM EDITOR

Alice Akunyili, M.D.
Kaplan Medical

Contents

Section Six: Appendix

USMLE® Step 2 Clinical Skills Exam

About the USMLE Step 2 Clinical Skills (CS) Exam

The 3-step USMLE examination required for medical licensure in the United States assesses a physician's ability to (a) apply knowledge, concepts, and principles, and (b) demonstrate fundamental patient-centered skills which constitute the basis of safe and effective patient care. Each of the 3 Steps complements the others.

Step 1 assesses whether one can understand and apply important concepts of the sciences basic to the practice of medicine. It is based on an integrated content outline which organizes basic science material along 2 dimensions: **system** and **process**. It is a 1-day multiple-choice exam.

Step 2 assesses whether one can apply medical knowledge, skills, and understanding of clinical science essential for the provision of patient care under supervision. It includes emphasis on health promotion and disease prevention. There are 2 components of Step 2.

- **Step 2 CK (Clinical Knowledge)** is based on an integrated content outline that organizes clinical science material along 2 dimensions: physician task and disease category. Step 2 CK uses a 1-day multiple-choice format to test clinical knowledge.

- **Step 2 CS (Clinical Skills)** is a "hands on" exam to test one's ability to gather information from patients, perform physical examinations, and communicate findings to patients and colleagues. The exam measures skills essential to patient care that cannot be measured by a traditional multiple-choice exam.

Step 3 assesses whether one can apply medical knowledge and understanding of biomedical and clinical science essential for the unsupervised practice of medicine, with emphasis on patient management in ambulatory settings. It is the final examination in the USMLE sequence.

EXAM OVERVIEW

Step 2 CS is a 1-day live examination which resembles a physician's typical workday in a clinic, doctor's office, ER, and/or hospital setting in the United States. The exam is administered at regional Clinical Skills Evaluation Centers (CSEC) in **Atlanta, Chicago, Houston, Philadelphia,** and **Los Angeles**.

- The focus of medical history you need to obtain in each case will be determined by the nature and complexity of the patient's presentation.

- Not every part of the history needs to be taken for every patient. Some patients will have acute problems while others will have more chronic ones.

- You will not have time to do a complete physical exam on every patient, nor is it necessary to do so. Pursue a focused physical examination based on the patient's complaint and information obtained during the history-taking.

Step 2 CS Strategy

It is impossible to conduct a full physical exam and obtain a lengthy patient history in 15 minutes. The key words for this time-critical task are **"pertinent history"** and **"focused physical examination."**

Note

Even though this is a simulated exam, make sure you perform physical examination maneuvers correctly and expect that some encounters may have positive physical findings. Accept any positive findings as real and factor them into your evolving physical diagnoses hypothesis.

The CS exam blueprint is designed to give you a fair representation of cases that a physician is likely to encounter in clinical settings in the United States. Examinees will be required to demonstrate clinical skills most comparable to the level of experience of a first-year medical resident.

Most cases are designed to test the type of history-taking and focused examination that demonstrates your ability to list and pursue plausible differential diagnoses in acute and non-acute situations. Some cases, however, may focus only on history-taking, physical exam, or counseling. Some scenarios, such as phone cases, may involve a parent of a child or a family member of an elderly patient who will not be present in the room. In these situations a physical examination of the patient will not be required; however, you will still be expected to take a history, counsel, articulate a differential diagnosis hypothesis and write a Patient Note (carefully read the doorway information instructions so you know the tasks that you are expected to perform!).

Clinical case categories include, but are not limited to:

• Cardiovascular	• Neurologic
• Elderly care	• Pediatric care
• Endocrine	• Preventive health
• Gastrointestinal	• Psychiatry
• Genitourinary	• Psychiatry
• Genitourinary	• Respiratory
• Musculoskeletal	• Women's health

EXAM SPECIFICS

The exam will include 12 patient encounters. (A very small number of non-scored patient encounters are included for research purposes, but those cases are integrated into the exam.)

- The Evaluation Center where the exam is given will simulate a healthcare environment comparable with a large medical clinic. When you enter the testing area, you will have 12 stations set up as fully equipped examination rooms.

- Each exam room door will post an instruction sheet ("doorway-information"), containing basic information about the case: patient's name, age, gender, reason for the visit, vital signs, and tasks that examinees are expected to perform.

- At the start of each encounter you will hear an announcement such as, *"Examinees you may begin your encounter."*

  - Read the instruction sheet, take notes on the scrap paper, knock on the door and begin your encounter, just as you would with a real patient. A second copy of the instruction sheet will be accessible in the exam room.

- You will conduct 12 examinations (15 minutes each) of a **"standardized patient"** (SP) chosen from a broad range of age and ethnic backgrounds, and trained to portray a patient with a high degree of reliability.

  - You must communicate with the SPs in a professional and empathetic manner, to establish a good doctor-patient rapport while simultaneously eliciting pertinent historic information and performing a focused physical examination.

  - You must address all the SPs concerns, explain and justify the diagnoses that are being considered, provide counseling when appropriate, inform and get the patient's agreement on planned diagnostic tests.

- After each encounter, you will have 10 minutes to record pertinent history and physical exam findings obtained during the encounter, to list diagnostic impressions (maximum of 3 in the order of likelihood) with support for each, and to outline the diagnostic studies planned.

Step 2 CS at a Glance

Total Exam Length:	8 hours including 2 breaks
Patient Encounters:	12
Length of Each Patient Encounter:	15 minutes
Time Allotted for Writing Each Patient Note:	10 minutes

STRATEGY AND TIME MANAGEMENT

Time management is critical during the CS exam, factoring in the success of your performance.

Patient Encounter: You will be expected to perform **15-minute** patient encounters for **12 SPs** during your exam.

- Each exam room door will have posted the patient's basic information (name, age, presenting complaint, pertinent vital signs, etc.); you must review this information before walking in.
- Assume all doorway information is accurate and use it when generating your differential diagnosis hypothesis.
- Typically, vital signs should not be repeated, but if you do repeat them, refer to the doorway information when developing your differential diagnosis.

Because the exam is standardized, all examinees receive the same information when they ask SPs the same or similar questions. The SPs you encounter during the exam are trained to document your actions in a fair and consistent manner. Immediately following each patient encounter, the SP fills out checklists to document questions you've asked, maneuvers you performed, and your demeanor and communication skills including proficiency with the English language during the encounter.

- Based on the patient's presenting complaint, doorway information, and additional information you obtain during the history, consider the most likely possible diagnoses and then explore the relevant ones as time permits.
- To monitor good time management, do the following:
  - During the patient interview, remember that your communication and interpersonal skills are evaluated based on your observable behaviors and your response to the patient's needs.
  - Demonstrate professionalism and good interpersonal/communication skills. Professionalism and public trust go hand-in-hand and they have been viewed as a way to improve patient care and preserve the doctor patient-relationship.
  - Address the patient in a clear manner; your English-proficiency is an equally important subcomponent of the CS exam.
  - Demonstrate appropriate clinical skills to obtain a competent history, conduct a focused physical exam, and generate a differential diagnosis and initial work-up using appropriate time management.

Note that certain parts of the physical exam must *not* be done: rectal, pelvic, genitourinary, female breast, corneal reflex, inguinal hernia, and throat swab. If you believe such exams are indicated, include them in the proposed diagnostic workup.

Patient Note: After each encounter, you will have **10 minutes** to record a complete Patient Note that should include:

- All relevant history taken
- Physical examinations performed
- Diagnostic impressions (in order of likelihood) and their supporting data
- Diagnostic workup for initial evaluation

Once you leave the exam room, you are not permitted to re-enter, so be sure you have obtained all necessary information before leaving. However, if you leave the patient encounter early, you can use the additional time to start your Patient Note. In the case of technical or administrative problems, typing the notes on the computer may not be an option. If that happens, you will be required to write your notes by hand. Therefore, be prepared to write one or more Patient Notes on the day of your exam. These notes need to be legible or they cannot be scored.

EXAM COMPONENTS

The CS exam is composed of 3 subcomponents:

- Communication and Interpersonal Skills (CIS)
- Spoken English Proficiency (SEP)
- Integrated Clinical Encounter (ICE)

CIS subcomponent assesses

- **Fostering the relationship**: listen attentively and show interest, care, concern, and respect
- **Gathering information**: establish chronology of the primary problem, identify patient concerns and assess impact of health issue on patient
- **Providing information**: explain the most likely diagnosis, encourage and answer questions
- **Helping the patient make decisions**: outline what should happen next linked to a rationale, assess patient's level of agreement and ability to carry out next steps
- **Supporting emotions**: seek clarification of patient's feelings to be sure you are correctly interpreting them, demonstrate understanding, empathy and support

SEP subcomponent assesses

- Clarity of spoken English communication within the doctor-patient encounter
- Frequency of pronunciation or word choice errors that affect comprehension
- Listener effort required to understand the examinees questions and responses
- Minimizing the need to repeat questions or statements

ICE subcomponent assesses

- **Data gathering** skills: patient information collected by history taking and physical examination reflecting your performance during the encounter as well as the documented summary of these findings in your Patient Note
- **Data interpretation** skills: completion of a Patient Note summarizing the findings of the patient encounter, diagnostic impression and justification, and patient diagnostic studies

EXAM SCORING

The Step 2 CS exam is a pass/fail exam. Examinees are scored in each of the 3 subcomponents: ICE, CIS, and SEP. **Examinees must pass each of the 3 subcomponents on the same day in order to pass.** Failure in one subcomponent will result in failure on the entire exam.

CIS subcomponent scoring

Checklists assessing your CIS performance based on observable behaviors are assessed by SPs on all 5 CIS subdivisions:

- Fostering the relationship
- Gathering information
- Providing information
- Helping the patient make decisions
- Supporting emotions

SEP subcomponent scoring

Standardized patients (SP) use rating scales to assess the examinees SEP performance.

ICE subcomponent scoring

- **History and Physical Examination checklists** scored by SPs
- **Global ratings** of **Patient Note** scored by trained physicians

A committee of clinicians and medical school clinical faculty develop the checklists.

For your score report, you will receive a Performance Profile covering the strengths and weaknesses of your performance across the 3 subcomponents. The Performance Profile is provided solely for your benefit; it will not be reported to any third parties.

USMLE STEP 2 CS PERFORMANCE PROFILE

	Lower Performance	Borderline Performance	Higher Performance
Integrated Clinical Encounter (ICE)			xxxxx*
Communication and Interpersonal Skills (CIS)			xxxxxxxxxxx
Spoken English Proficiency (SEP)			xxxxxxx

"Borderline performance" is an approximate representation of where the scores of high failures and low passers would fall in the profile. The width of the bands is based upon the idea of measurement precision, and is intended to reflect the approximate variation in scores, both higher and lower, that would be expected to occur if an examinee were tested repeatedly using compatible sets of Clinical Skills cases.

If a subcomponent is failed but the band of X's extends beyond the "borderline performance" area, this does not reflect a mistake in scoring; it indicates a relatively high failing performance.

ON TEST DAY

The CS exam begins with an onsite orientation explaining use of the diagnostic equipment available in the exam rooms, test rules, and test procedures. Be sure not to miss this session. At the orientation you will have the opportunity to ask questions.

- The exam lasts about 8 hours, which includes one 30-minute break (after the 5th encounter) and one 15-minute break (after the 9th encounter).
- A light meal is provided. You may bring your own food, provided that no refrigeration or preparation is required.
- There are vending machines for drinks.

We strongly encourage you to review the orientation video in advance available on the USMLE website. In addition, we recommend the following:

- Arrive at the test center 30 minutes before the scheduled exam.
- Bring your Scheduling Permit and the Confirmation notice.
- An unexpired government-issued form of identification (driver's license or passport) that also has your signature. If the names printed on the 2 documents are different (except for middle names), contact USMLE well ahead of Test Day. Without acceptable level of identification you will not be permitted to take the test.
- Wear comfortable, professional clothing, and a clean white lab or clinic coat.
- Bring an unenhanced standard stethoscope.
- Keep your wallet and driver license in your pant or coat pocket at all times.

OTHER POINTS TO NOTE

- Wearing a watch is prohibited during CS exam; a clock is on the wall inside of each patient room, enabling you to follow your time.

- Each exam center contains a locked storage area with small cubicles for storage of necessary personal items; you will be restricted from that area for the entire exam, including breaks.

- Once the on-site orientation has started, you may not leave that area until the exam is over.

- You may not discuss the cases with your fellow examinees at any time.

- Conversation among examinees and with patients in any language other than English is prohibited at all times.

- Proctors will monitor all examinee activity.

- On the day of the exam, you may be asked to sign documents intended to confirm your understanding and willingness to abide by USMLE policies and procedures. You may also be asked to complete demographic and feedback surveys after the exam.

Communication and Interpersonal Skills (CIS)

Communication and Interpersonal Skills (CIS)

2

The patient–physician relationship should be the center and focus of all clinical medicine. Excellent communication skills have been shown to improve patient outcomes, patient satisfaction, as well as physician satisfaction. Contrary to the beliefs of some physicians, using more appropriate skills does not prolong the encounter. These skills can be learned if sufficient time is dedicated to practice and feedback.

Effective communication on the exam will allow you to efficiently obtain the information needed during the brief encounter. Expect the standardized patients (SPs) to respond in a realistic way within the confines of their behavioral profiles. The type of responses you receive will sometimes depend on your own personality and characteristics. Following the cooperative responses of the patient, you can determine which body systems to focus on during the physical exam (PE). The patient will become less anxious and more compliant with your requests when you give clear instructions, explain what you are doing each step of the way, and assure the patient that each maneuver is medically important.

Likewise, in closing the encounter, summarize your findings from the history, confirming their accuracy with the patient. Pertinent findings from the PE might be mentioned in the summary as well. Answering any questions the patient may have also gives you a final opportunity to reinforce your competency. Finally, armed with adequate positive and negative findings from the history and physical, you will be able to produce the patient note more quickly, with better organization, and with greater accuracy.

The communication skills, along with the PE, are scored by an SP who checks off items on a computerized list as soon as you leave the room. The CIS score is an *average* of the 12 scored encounters; therefore, you could perform awkwardly or ineffectively in 1 or 2 encounters yet still succeed on the exam.

Using the interpersonal skills checklist, the SP rates your skills in interviewing and collecting information, counseling and delivering information, establishing rapport, and maintaining a positive personal manner. Each skill area involves a handful of key characteristics that are important for effective communication in general. Mastery in each area can be achieved by plenty of practice. To deepen and expand self-awareness, seek feedback from the role-playing patient regarding his perception of your interpersonal skills.

TIMING THE PATIENT ENCOUNTER

Time management on the Step 2 CS is crucial. For encounters that require both a history and physical examination, we recommend that you spend up to 1 minute outside the room reviewing the doorway information. Spend 6–7 minutes greeting the patient, eliciting the chief complaint, history of present illness (HPI), and relevant past medical history (PMH), asking about any visible physical findings and related review of systems. Spend 15–30 seconds hand-washing, and then take 3-4 minutes to perform a focused physical exam. Finally, take 3-4 minutes to explain to the patient your findings, counsel, address concerns, and answer any questions.

Note

For each encounter on the exam, you will get a warning that only 5 minutes remain. You should be in the middle of performing the PE when you get this announcement.

1 min	• Read doorway information; copies are in the room and adjacent to the desk where you write the note
	• Start thinking of a differential diagnosis list, and write down several of the most likely ones. Jot down a mnemonic if needed.
	• Knock and enter patient room
At 7 1/2 min	• End interview (critical point) including writing down key points. This written information will ensure accurate and thorough notes.
From 7 1/2–8 min	• Wash hands and start examination
	• Continue the history-taking during the PE
At 11 1/2 min	• End PE and if needed, write down key points. This written information will ensure accurate and thorough notes.
From 11 1/2–15 min	• Do closing including counseling and end the visit
From 15–25 min	• Write note

Note

A wall clock is present in each room; you may want to write the time of entry so you can keep track of the critical time points noted in the table. Pacing yourself is very important for a higher test score.

EVALUATION OF CIS

The following pages present a detailed description of the evaluation of interpersonal and communication skills.

1. Knocked before entering

Knock before going into the examining room. By knocking first, you alert the patient that someone is about to enter. Knocking is a first step in building trust and showing respect. Knock 3 times, wait 3 seconds, open the door and then enter the room. Do not be timid. Even if you are unsure that you heard the SP say "come in," enter after 3 seconds. Do not hesitate and waste valuable time.

Credit will always be given if you knock. In some cases the SP has been trained to NOT respond to the knock, to see if you will enter or just keep knocking (factors which will affect your use of time and also the relationship).

2. Introduction—used last name and title

Set a tone of friendliness and positive rapport by making a cordial introduction. You will be given credit for introducing yourself by name, greeting the patient by name and for identifying your role in the hospital.

- It is proper to introduce yourself using title, first, and last name or title and last name alone. Choose either Dr. Susan Smith or Dr. Smith.
- Never refer to yourself or to a patient by first name only.
- Remain aware of words you are using during all phases of the interview. It is often disquieting to patients if physicians use statements that are too informal, and it may detract from professionalism.
  - If there is any ambiguity in your role, such as your status as a student, explain your relation to the patient's care. If appropriate, you can refer to yourself as a senior medical student or resident on service.

- Many patients will be comfortable receiving a handshake upon introduction. Shake hands if you feel comfortable doing so. A welcoming handshake can serve to relax an anxious patient.
  - However, this form of greeting may not always be appropriate. If a patient is in discomfort, distress, or severe pain, offering a handshake during introduction may not be appropriate. Instead, focus on the patient's comfort by offering to help him move to a more comfortable position.

> Establish eye contact with the SP before you introduce yourself. If you do extend your hand and he does not take it, do not force him to shake. Just withdraw your hand and continue your introduction. Always take your cue from the SP. It shows how well you are focused and paying attention.

3. Established patient's preferred title

Address all patients as "Mr," or "Ms," or "Dr" if they have an advanced degree such as an M.D., a D.D.S. or PhD. Then confirm that this is their preferred title.

- Do not use first names only unless the patient requests that you do so. Referring to a patient using a level of formality lower than the level used to refer to yourself would place the patient in an unequal and inferior position.
  - The exception would be a case of an adolescent or child; in that case it is acceptable to use a first name. If you are unsure about the pronunciation of your patient's name, always confirm that you pronounced it correctly.

> Ask the SP what she would prefer to be called or how to pronounce her name if needed. Make sure to use her name periodically throughout the encounter.

4. Clarified role

Explain to the patient your role and your understanding of why the patient has come to be seen by a doctor. This statement informs the patient what will be occurring during the 15-minute encounter.

- For example, "Hello Mr/Ms Jones. I'm Dr. Smith, the clinic or emergency room physician assigned to your care today. I understand you have come here because you xxxxxx (could have pain, are returning for follow-up or annual check-up, want to get test results, are trying to determine if your treatment is working). I will be asking you some questions and examining you, and then discussing my findings and impressions with you."

It is also helpful to align the patient and your expectations about the encounter.

- For example, "Is that your expectation as well?" or "Is that correct?"

This is also a good opportunity to acknowledge that you will be taking notes on important details of the history and physical exam. This will ensure accurate recording of all pertinent information and will help in writing a good patient note.

To help establish rapport, start the interaction by asking how the patient is doing today.

- For example, "How are you feeling right now?" If the patient previously had a change in the treatment plan (started a new medication, started on a diet), you can add that to your inquiry. "How have you been doing since you started on x?"

5. Had professional appearance in dress, grooming, and hygiene

A physician's appearance can influence the success of an interview. Patients have an image of what they expect regarding the appearance of a clinician. If you meet those expectations it will build confidence in your medical abilities. Patients form their first impression of you based on your appearance as you enter the room.

- Surveys show patients prefer medical personnel to dress in white coats and wear shoes instead of sneakers. Make sure your white coat is clean and neat.

- Wear comfortable, conservative clothing. It is suggested that men wear trousers, a dress shirt, a tie, and dark shoes, while women wear slacks or a skirt, low-heeled and closed-toe shoes, and conservative jewelry.

- Avoid wearing jeans, sneakers, or sandals.

- Pull your hair back away from your face, trim your nails, and use no products with scents (such as hairspray, perfume, or cologne). You would never want to initiate any allergic reaction in your SP.

- Make sure there are no body or mouth odors or stale clothing odors.

Professional appearance shows that you take pride in yourself, which instills the SP's confidence in you.

---

6. Showed care and concern for patient

- It is important to create an impression that you truly care about the patient. Your overall goal must be to put the patient at ease and diminish the level of anxiety present at the onset of the encounter. This can be accomplished with both verbal and non-verbal (body language).

- Besides choosing appropriate words and phrases, attempt to use a facial expression, posture and tone of voice that conveys the same message of concern.
  - Look directly at the patient (especially when patient is talking).
  - Avoid writing voluminous notes while conversing.
  - Do not stand during the interview/discussion, because it can make the patient feel you are controlling instead of partnering with him or her.
  - Keep an appropriate distance from the patient so you are not too close but also are not across the room.
  - Make sure to appropriately respond to what your patient is saying. If he is talking about losing a job or loved one, sharing that he is in pain, acknowledge your concern and empathy with a statement such as, "I'm so sorry" or "That must be very difficult."

- Patients should leave feeling they had a physician who cared. Typically, patient satisfaction is positively impacted more by a caring concerned physician that created a welcoming atmosphere than by medical competence.

- Poor positioning may be a sign of discomfort. Ask the patient, "What can I do to make you more comfortable?"
  - If you notice the patient is displaying a negative emotion such as sitting with slumped shoulders and a sad face, acknowledge that you have noticed and are concerned. Say, "I am concerned that something is bothering you. I can't help but notice you look unhappy. Is there something you would like to share with me?" and "I know it may be difficult to open up to a doctor you just met, but I want to help you in any way I can."

- Talking with the patient during the physical exam will reduce her anxiety and increase cooperation. Tell her what you are going to do (e.g., examine the ears), and at times, why (e.g., to look for redness). Proceeding through the physical exam without speaking to the patient will create unnecessary tension and there will be a loss of credit. Maintain eye contact while you are examining the patient so you can determine if anything you are doing is causing her pain or embarrassment.

- You may ask additional questions while performing the physical exam if you are able to maintain eye contact while doing so. However, be careful.

  - For example, asking patients if they have ever had heart trouble when you have just finished listening to the heart, or asking about a family history of cancer after completing a lung exam, may sound scary. Instead, state at the beginning of the physical exam, "As I examine parts of your body, I may ask you some standard questions related to that area. Please do not think that I have found something wrong."

- During the physical exam, be careful of facial expressions or gestures such as a frown that may communicate something is wrong. Patients will often be watching your face for information. A caring expression and tone of voice goes a long way to put patients at ease.

- Never alarm patients unnecessarily. When asking certain questions such as "Have you ever been tested for HIV/AIDS?," mention that certain questions are routine. Without sufficient information and confirmation, never suggest a catastrophic diagnosis as part of your conclusion.

- Be careful of how you ask a question but also of *when* it is asked. Confronting a difficult subject such as domestic violence too early in an encounter can be inappropriate. Timing is everything.

  - Finding a late point in the history has the advantage of having given you time to establish rapport with the patient and show your skills at expressing empathy and reassurance. In order to be comfortable enough to open up to you on this difficult subject, patients must truly believe you understand and care.

- Washing your hands in the exam room is another way to show you are concerned about a patient's health. Your cleanliness will protect them from any infectious disease process that could be transmitted from another patient.

  - You will also be given credit if you choose to use gloves. However, wearing gloves creates an unnecessary barrier between you and the patient and therefore consider using hand washing as your first choice. Resort to gloves only if you have a lesion on your own hands that you do not want to transmit to the patient. If so, be sure to verbalize your reason for this decision.

As you work through the PE, the SP will always feel more comfortable when you talk, letting her know what you plan to do. It's startling to be touched without warning, even if it's a gesture of empathy.

- For example, on a past CS exam an SP played a patient who couldn't open her eyes because of light sensitivity. The doctor touched the patient's hand to reassure her, but he didn't let her know in advance. As a result, the SP was startled and afraid. Had the doctor given a warning, the SP would have perceived that gesture of empathy in a positive way.

7. Displayed confident manner and rapport

Always project an image of both confidence and competence throughout the encounter. Patients should feel that you are comfortable in your role as a physician in charge. Things which reflect a lack of confidence include unnecessary pauses during the history or physical examination and repetitively asking, "Is that okay?" Also, talking very fast, tapping your foot, or saying "ummm" can make you appear nervous or insecure.

You are expected to interact with an SP as you would with any real patient, i.e., demonstrate purposeful exploration of relevant components of both the history and physical exam. You will not have time to do a complete physical examination on every patient, only a targeted one. Perform the exam with confidence, being aware and attentive to patient discomfort and modesty. Avoid appearing timid, tentative, unsure, or awkward, and demonstrate a gentle nature.

Remember that the SPs are well trained to mimic the chosen illnesses. This training includes exposure to a very detailed description of the relevant history and physical examination required for each individual case. So in order to appear competent, you must ask the correct types of questions and select the appropriate components of the physical examination.

8. Had respectful and nonjudgmental attitude

Passing judgment on the patient may result in your being considered an unsuitable listener. It is not your role to judge on any patient behaviors such as the use of alcohol and illicit drugs. Your job is to gather the data that will help you make a correct assessment. Showing sensitivity does not mean that you approve of the behavior. If the patient appears uncomfortable, recognize her discomfort and normalize it. "I know discussing these issues can be uncomfortable; however, it is important to know this information for every patient. Is there something I can do to help you feel more comfortable?"

Judgment can be reflected in your choice of words, body language and even the tone of your voice. Don't ask questions in the negative, such as, "You don't use drugs, do you?" Don't look shocked or surprised if you hear a disturbing answer, and don't raise your eyebrows or frown. Reactions that portray disgust or disapproval will block communication. Be sensitive to all the messages you are sending and control them as best you can. Make sure your facial expression remains consistently respectful.

- It is not necessary to respond after every answer.
- Avoid antagonistic phrases like "You do or did what?" which imply judgment, especially when the question concerns the patient's lifestyle.
- A simple "thank you" or "okay" is often sufficient when the patient is giving information. These responses establish an open, safe atmosphere.
- Reserve all patient education for the end of the encounter.
- Never contradict or impose your standards on the patient. As a rule patients like to respond to questions in a way that attempts to satisfy the physician in order to gain approval. If they perceive that a certain type of answer consistently meets with your approval and another type does not, they may stop providing honest answers to your questions.

Don't move or touch underwear, bras or even gowns, unless requested to do so by the patient, and never touch without explaining first. This applies to draping the patient, untying the hospital gown and doing anything on the physical examination. Explain what you are doing during every stage of the examination with statements such as "I am going to press on your knee" or "I need to listen to your chest".

> Stay and respond in a neutral manner. If the SP senses judgment, she may not answer your questions truthfully for fear of judgment.

9. Focused attention and concentration on patient

The best way to stay calm under pressure is to focus your attention solely on the patient, and not let yourself be distracted by anything connected to yourself. During the entire 15 minutes you spend with the SP, all you should be doing is establishing a rapport, obtaining sufficient information to generate a diagnostic hypothesis, and considering a plan for how to validate it. Pay close attention to everything the patient says and does. Everything is there for a reason.

During the Step 2 CS exam, take every bit of evidence as a clue. A bandaged wrist may suggest intimate partner violence; a bruise on the upper arm of an elderly patient may indicate elder abuse or a recent fall. If a patient coughs into a handkerchief, ask to see the sputum; hemoptysis may be noted. Remember, the SP will not usually volunteer the very piece of information that could guide your clinical reasoning in a new direction. You will need to be a careful observer. Ask open-ended questions so you don't get a limited answer and miss information. For example:

- Asking if the patient has ever been hospitalized does not mean you are asking if the patient ever had surgery. Surgery can be outpatient and the patient may not assume this is a hospitalization.

- Asking if the patient has any allergies may not reveal a food or seasonal allergy; he may think you only mean an allergy to medications.

- Asking if the patient is on any medications, he may not relay over-the-counter medications because they weren't not prescribed.

Watch for indications of discomfort from body language such as poor positioning or evidence of pain. Improving the position of the patient may impact your data gathering score. If the patient is more comfortable it will be easier to elicit a good history in a timely fashion. Continue to consider the patient's comfort during the course of the interview. You can make your patient more comfortable by raising or lowering the back of the examining table as needed, by extending the leg rest or by helping a change in position.

It is key to look at patients when asking questions, giving them your full attention. This will give the impression that you care about them and what is going on with them. In any performance situation, it's possible to become extremely self-conscious and lose focus on the patient. If you become distracted and miss what the patient says, you can say "I'm sorry, could you repeat that? I'm not sure I got it."

Several things may indicate that your attention has wandered from the patient. You may lose points if your eyes wander as you think of your next several questions, if you proceed too slowly or quickly, or if you constantly look at the clock. Do not spend too much time on the clipboard taking notes in excess of that which is necessary. And never leave the patient unnecessarily exposed. To auscultate the heart, for instance, do not raise the gown up from the waist and expose the entire torso; lower the gown instead from the top, exposing only the upper chest and shoulders.

Finally, never assume that anything is so obvious that it does not need to be acknowledged. Any makeup that is used must always be acknowledged. The SP may use appropriate colors to represent trauma, infection, jaundice or anemia. If you do not verbalize your findings it is as if you did not see what is present and you will lose points on this skill.

An SP will never try to trick you; everything he does is for a reason. Pay attention and he will guide you through the encounter.

- For example if an SP is wearing socks and all of your other patients were barefoot, there is a reason; find out why. If you need to untie the SP's gown, be sure to retie it before moving on. Make your patient's comfort your priority.

10. Listened attentively without interrupting

If a patient doesn't immediately answer a question you have asked, wait in silence for patients to think about the answers to your questions and sometimes to process their feelings. Once speaking, patients' answers should not be cut off. Let them finish speaking, even if there are pauses and silences. Interrupting disrupts their train of thought. Quietly wait for each answer to be completed and don't fill in words for the patient. Grant them the proper respect of being heard fully. If the question has hit on a sensitive issue and the patient becomes teary, offer a tissue, sit down, and quietly wait. In general, a brief pause or silence will encourage patients to say more. Silence is one of the least invasive interviewing techniques, one that encourages the patient to open up and share more freely. However, if the silence becomes prolonged observe for signs of distress since a prolonged silence may be indicative of distress and you can address this by recognizing the patient's distress and your role in causing it. You could state, "You seem distressed and I'm so sorry that my questions have upset you. This information is important, so is there anything I can do to assist you or should we come back to this a little later?"

Don't worry about the lack of time in a sensitive case like grieving or depression; never lose sight of the human connection. The Step 2 CS exam is primarily a test of interpersonal and communication skills. Step 2 CS cases are carefully planned to take approximately 15 minutes, including any expression of emotion or hesitation on the part of the SP.

Of course, at times, it may be necessary to interrupt patients. They may be talking on and on about irrelevant matters, such as a problem a family member may be having. In such cases, you can gain the patients' trust even more strongly by firmly interrupting to refocus on them. Cut in whenever patients hesitate slightly, look them straight in the eyes, and say, "Excuse me for interrupting, Ms. Jones." Next, acknowledge whatever the patient was talking about by stating, "I know these concerns have really been troubling you, and we can discuss them at a follow-up visit." Then bring the focus back to the patient: "However, right now I want to focus completely on you." Chances are they will feel validated that someone cares enough to want to focus on their symptoms.

Avoid repeating the same question, unless for clarification. If you are unsure what a patient has said or think an answer is vague, ask the question again, explaining that you are trying to verify that you heard correctly. Sometimes patients will answer the same question using different words and therefore the meaning will be clearer.

Occasionally there may be an inconsistency between a fact stated later in the history compared to an earlier stated fact. Therefore you may need to ask for clarification to be sure you have obtained the correct information.

Never quickly repeat a question before the SP has had time to respond. It may appear that you don't care whether the response is accurate–just that it is given rapidly.

Learn to feel comfortable with silence. When you give the SP time to think and respond, she feels respected and heard. SPs are very aware of 15 minutes; they have been trained to think and to hesitate in responding to see if you will interrupt. At the same time, however, they will not impede you from completing your encounter in the allotted 15 minutes. An SP may speed up or shorten responses, but she will always include all the information you asked for as long as she is not interrupted.

11. Maintained comfortable eye contact

Position yourself so that the patient can easily see you without straining. Attempt to maintain your eyes as close as possible to being at the same level as those of the patient. If the patient is lying down facing either right or left, move around to that side of the table and sit down at a slight angle so that patients do not need to extend their necks. Sitting down is considered a positive behavior by American patients because it projects time to listen and concentrate.

When you encounter patients lying on their backs, remember to stand but also at a slight angle.

Patients should not have to turn their heads to see you. Never stand behind the patient during the history or the closing. If the patient is sitting at the end of the table, sitting down would be less intimidating and would help create a better initial rapport between you and the patient.

In general, if you seem to be avoiding eye contact or look distracted, you will not be seen as listening to or caring about the patient. Comfortable eye contact reinforces a sense of trust and credibility. If you shift your eyes around the room or avoid looking directly at the patient, you may communicate a lack of self-confidence.

Even during physical examination eye contact remains important. For example, you may need to observe the patient's face for any signs of pain or discomfort.

> Staring at the SP will make him feel awkward and uncomfortable. He would prefer you to look and listen with interest and concern, without staring into his eyes or at a specific body part.

12. Maintained comfortable and appropriate distance

Standing too close or too far away may suggest either a stance of aggression or timidity, respectively. As a general rule, 2 feet is about right for personal proximity in the American culture. Observe for cues from the SP. If the patient continuously leans back, you are probably too close. If the patient leans forward, you are probably too far. It is appropriate to stand closer to a patient suffering from bilateral hearing loss.

13. Used proper draping technique

Many patients will already be covered to the waist with the drape. If not already on the patient, the drape sheet may be folded on the stool in the examining room. Before you begin the medical interview, reach for the drape, unfold it halfway, and place it immediately on the patient from the waist down. Before covering the patient say "I'd like to cover you now to make you feel a little more comfortable." That way, you are indirectly asking for permission and showing empathy for the patient's comfort. You can also encourage the patient to adjust the drape to maximize his own comfort.

- Strictly speaking, as long as you drape the patient no later than the beginning of the physical exam, you should receive credit. However, it is preferable to do so at the beginning of the history since the drape is on the stool upon which you will be sitting. It makes logical sense to do it first since you won't want to sit on the drape you will be using later. The one exception to this general rule is that any patient lying down must be draped even before beginning the history.

As soon as you have completed examining a particular section of the body, replace the drape without delay. Also if part of the examination involves asking the patient to stand, replace the drape after the patient returns to the table.

Regarding the hospital gown, prior to beginning the physical examination, create a mutually agreed upon plan with the patient. Some patients will prefer to have the physician untie, retie, raise and lower the gown, some will prefer to do those things themselves, and some will prefer to share the hospital gown responsibilities. Whatever decision is made will hold for the entire physical exam and the issue will not have to be discussed again during each portion of the exam.

> The drape is not just for covering your SP; it gives you the opportunity to really see your patient. You are covering him and focusing on him. Observe his physical, mental, and emotional demeanor. This moment may tell you more than the doorway scenario.

14. Non-verbal communication

There are various ways to show patients that, as their physician, you are focused on what they are saying and want to hear more.

- Nod your head
- Lean in toward the patient
- Use sufficient short pauses and at times, use long appropriate silences
- Maintain an engaged listening posture
- Do not cross your arms or place your hands in your pockets

15. Elicited chief complaint (CC)

One method is to begin the history with an open-ended question such as, "What caused you to come see me today?" An alternative approach would be to repeat the chief complaint stated in the doorway information and then verify that it is the chief complaint.

- "My nurse told me you came here today for [CC]. Is that correct?
- "I would like to hear in your own words what has been bothering you."

For most cases the CC stated in the doorway information will be the same complaint stated by the patient in the room. However, on occasion, the patient may have not been comfortable telling the intake person the actual complaint since it may have felt too private. That patient may have found it difficult to disclose the real complaint to anyone besides the physician. For these cases, the patient may change the CC from the one stated on the door.

- A 60-year-old man suffering from erectile dysfunction may initially state to the nurse an unrelated urinary or gastrointestinal complaint, but then tell the physician about his sexual dysfunction

16. Established timeline of chief complaint (CC)

- The patient must feel that the physician is attempting to elicit as much background information as possible regarding the chief complaint and to understand what may be causing it to occur. The SP will not necessarily be looking for specific questions but rather for the presence of a thought process that uses characteristics of the complaint as well as other associated symptoms and their timing in relation to the chief complaint. The physician is not being graded on a specific history checklist as part of data gathering but rather on an overall impression created on the SP that reflects the ability to do a logical targeted history.

17. Asked open-ended questions

Open-ended questions are those that require a sentence or two describing something in the patient's own words and encourage a longer, more detailed response. They do not limit the response the patient can provide. Begin with general open ended questions to enable patients to tell you as much as they want about the current problem. For example "What caused you to come see me today?" This allows them to begin with their own narrative. Then proceed to more directed open- ended ones to help focus the questioning. For example, "What makes your pain worse?"

You can also end your history with one last open- ended question such as "Is there anything else you would like to tell me about your health that we did not discuss?"

> When you do not use open-ended questions, the SP does not feel encouraged to tell her story. She will merely answer yes or no without any detail.

18. Followed up with close-ended questions

Close-ended questions will be answered with a simple yes/no or a few words. Close-ended questions will fill in specific details not already provided by the patient. If asked too early, relevant information may be lost. For example, if your case is about a patient with lower abdominal pain, you should have in mind some associated symptoms by the time the initial history questions have been answered. Asking "Do you have diarrhea?" or "Have you been feeling nauseated?" will yield a more direct answer than "Do you have any other symptoms?" If asked that way the SP would probably say, "Like what?" Typically at the end of the history of present illness, closed ended questions will help you identify patterns of symptoms characteristic of the common diseases tested on the CS exam. In addition, most questions regarding past medical history will be asked as closed-ended ones.

A fine balance can be struck between these two types of questioning. Proceed from the more general to the more specific ones. That way, patients will initially be able to express what is important to them and you will still be able to obtain detailed, significant and accurate data in a timely fashion.

> Asking about "change"—any change in sleep, diet, bowel habits, etc.—saves time and lets the SP tell the story. Closed-ended questions should logically follow from open-ended questions (thus, use no non-sequitors). When done this way, the SP will find it easy to follow your line of questioning.

19. Used non-leading questions

Questions should be stated in a neutral manner to avoid leading the patient into answering in a way that compromises accuracy. Neutrality is achieved by using the affirmative mode, rather than the negative: "Mr. Brown, have you ever used tobacco products?" instead of "You don't smoke, do you?" "Any nausea or vomiting?" instead of "No nausea or vomiting?" Questions should be asked in a way that encourages patients to answer candidly without fear of being judged or blamed for behaviors that can compromise their health, such as smoking cigarettes. If you were to say to a patient "You don't smoke, do you?" the patient might be uneasy about revealing the true history.

Be careful about leading your patients down a path framed from your own assumptions. For example, ask a patient with vaginal bleeding and clots "What did the clot look like?" rather than "Did the clot look like a piece of liver?" Your concept of a piece of liver may be based primarily on size while that of the patient may be based on texture. In other words, you may be asking if it was a large smooth clot, while the patient who responds yes may be telling you just that the blood looked smooth. If allowed to describe the clot to you, the same patient may say "It looked like a grape" which would reflect a much smaller clot.

20. Asked clear and concise questions

It is important to ask only one question at a time. Ask the question, then pause and wait for an answer before going on to the next one. Don't barrage the patient with a string of questions. Too often physicians run questions together in a list. "Has anyone in your family ever had high blood pressure, high cholesterol, strokes, or any heart condition that you know of?" "Have you had any nausea, vomiting, constipation or diarrhea?" Separate these items and ask them one at a time. Otherwise, the patient will become confused and feel rushed. Out of a sense of sheer confusion the patient may simply say no.

In addition, you will have used poor time management by running questions together in this way. The SP will probably say, "What? Which one?" and then you will have to start all over again. Worse yet, the SP may respond only to the final question in a string of questions, thus misleading you into thinking that the answer applies to all the previous parts as well and thereby undermining your clinical reasoning.

Asking questions without giving the patient an opportunity to answer interferes with clear communication. However, it is acceptable to use a list of questions if the choices are mutually exclusive and there is only one correct choice from the entire list. For example, you can ask your patient "Are your sexual partners male, female or both?" It is also acceptable to ask simple combination questions of 2 items routinely grouped together such as, "Any nausea or vomiting?" "Any tingling or numbness?" or "Any fever or chills?"

> When asked several questions at a time, the SP has been trained to answer only the last one with a simple "yes" or "no." The result: you may be misled.

21. Paraphrased and checked-in with the patient

All through the encounter, briefly either repeat back or rephrase a patient's key words based on your understanding of the stated facts. Repeating back the last few words of a sentence, echoing, and then pausing, will encourage your patient to give you more details. Interpreting what you just heard will not only show the patient that you are listening but will also provide an opportunity to correct any wrong information.

Shortly after discussing the chief complaint (by having asked, "What caused you to come in today?") and obtaining answers to a few other follow-up questions, it is a good idea to reflect the main points to the patient. Afterward, ask, "Is that correct?" If you've misunderstood any part of the response, the patient can then clarify. Paraphrasing will assist you greatly in your clinical reasoning. You need not repeat back the exact statement of the patient but rather your interpretation that reflects that you understood both the content and meaning of the statement.

Here are some examples of reflection and paraphrasing:

Doctor: "I see you're wearing an Ace bandage on your wrist. What happened there?"

Patient: "Oh, I hurt my wrist playing pool yesterday."

Doctor: (Nodding) "Playing polo?"

Patient: "No, no—playing pool."

Doctor: "Oh, okay. Playing pool."

Doctor: "Have you had any change in your weight lately?"

Patient: "Yeah, I've lost about 7 or 8 pounds."

Doctor: "Over what period of time?"

Patient: "Let's see—over about the past 2 months."

Doctor: "So, you were in good health until 2 months ago when you began to lose weight, is that correct?"

Doctor: "Has your weight changed lately?"

Patient: "Yes, I must have lost about 7 or 8 pounds."

Doctor: "Over what length of time?"

Patient: "About 2 months."

Doctor: "So you've lost about 7 or 8 pounds over the past 2 weeks?"

Patient: "No, not 2 weeks; it's been about 2 months."

Doctor: "Oh, 2 months. All right."

Finally, remember that paraphrasing provides you with a good opportunity to take a few notes. Since you initially are not gathering any new information, a break in eye contact will be accepted by the patient.

> When you paraphrase information back to the SP, even if it's just a phrase such as "vomited once, no blood," the SP feels heard. It also gives the SP the opportunity to make sure you are both 'on the same page.'

22. Elicited additional, including hidden concerns

In order for patients to leave the encounter satisfied, all their concerns must be identified and addressed. The patient will not always openly volunteer this information. Many concerns remain hidden and will only come out when a dedicated physician probes for all of them. You must help patients achieve their specific goals in seeking medical care.

Not every patient with the same chief complaint has the same hidden concerns. These concerns result from an individual's unique history and past exposures. One patient with abdominal pain may fear cancer as a result of having a family member with similar pain who was diagnosed with cancer. Another patient may fear surgery as a result of having undergone a prior surgical procedure that resulted in multiple post-operative complications. To address these varying concerns the physician must be aware of them. Therefore, always ask patients "What worries you the most about your CC?"

Another category of hidden concerns relate to family history. Many patients fear that they too are either at risk of or in the process of developing the same diseases that plagued other family members. This is especially true if they personally viewed the day to day difficulties the family member experienced or if they were present when that family member succumbed to the disease. Therefore, it is important to also identify these hidden concerns.

> A clue of some kind will usually be given by the SP that there is a hidden concern which should be addressed. This clue could be a verbal comment, a change in tone or speech pattern an emotional reaction, or a simple shift in physical presence. Stay focused on your patient and you will witness the change in demeanor.

23. Asked about impact on patient's life

Ask directly how the presenting symptom has affected the patient's daily activities, family or work. The symptom may have impacted the patient in a physical, psychological or social way. Obviously a more long-standing complaint will have had the opportunity to more significantly impact the life of the patient. However, even a complaint that only began several hours prior to presentation may have already affected the patient. One patient may have been in the process of completing a major work project with a deadline that evening and had to leave work to seek care. Another patient may be a single parent and was at home caring for two small children and could not find anyone to watch them and therefore had to bring these children to the emergency room. Knowing the specific impact on any individual enables the physician to address the concerns and needs specific to that patient.

> No matter how minor the chief complaint, it will have an impact on the life of the patient (even if it's just a matter of the time taken to come to the clinic).

24. Asked what patient thought was going on

Prior to delivering the diagnostic impression, it is recommended to ask the patient, "What do you think is causing your symptom?" Care must be taken to ask this question in the proper context so as not to receive an answer from the patient such as, "Why are you asking me that? You are the physician."

Be sure to explain to the patient the reason for your question.

- "I want to be sure that I address any concerns you may have and correct any misinformation you may have obtained from the media or other sources. I also want to be sure that I provide you with enough information to fully understand the probable cause of your symptom and to meet your expectations of this visit."
  - Attempt to see the presenting complaint through the eyes of the patient and understand the patient's perspective.

> Patients are smart and they have the internet. They will always have an idea of 'what's going on' with them, whether they tell you or not. Ask them what they think.

25. Used lay language or offered explanation

Patients should be regarded as knowing very little about the meaning of specialized medical terminology, so be sure to choose words and phrases that they will easily understand. Use language which any speaker of English can understand, with or without a specialized education. Furthermore, never undermine a positive rapport with the patient by showing off your technical expertise using medical jargon.

Medical jargon can easily creep into conversation. This is especially true if the word seems commonplace to you, such as trauma, hypertension, or CT scan.

- If you accidentally use a technical or medical term, explain immediately what it means in simple, straightforward language. The SP will give credit on this basis.
  - If you use medical terminology without explaining or if the patient has to ask what a term means, credit will not be given.

When preparing for your CS exam, be sure that you are able to describe in plain language what is going on in the patient's body and what tests you will be ordering. Never assume that patients will understand even simple medical terms such as hypertension that have become part of everyday speech.

- Patients may not tell you they don't understand a term you used, and will leave the encounter without being fully informed.

When you use medical jargon without explaining in simpler terms, the SP may feel inferior and even stupid. She may hesitate to ask for an explanation, which could cause her to leave with incorrect information. If you use medical terms, always clarify what they mean.

26. Incorporated appropriate use of continuers

Many short phrases and statements exist which inform patients that you, as the physician, would like to hear more information on a particular subject. They will typically encourage the patient to continue speaking. Learn to incorporate some of these statements into your clinical encounters.

- "I see"
- "Uh-huh, go on"
- "Mm-hmm"
- "Tell me more"
- "Yes, and then"

27. Incorporated appropriate use of transitions

Transitions (i.e., transitional words and phrases) are like signposts, alerting patients that you have obtained sufficient information on the current subject and are ready to move to a new area of questioning. For example, they will signal that you are moving from the history to the PE, and then to the closing.

- Transitional statements allow patients to follow along with the logic of your inquiry and thus keep the communication clear. By conveying an impression of orderly thinking, transitions will foster confidence and trust in your judgment.
- Increase sensitivity by always including a transition before embarking on the components of the personal social history and reminding and reassuring patients that what they will now tell you will be kept confidential. At this point you can also say to the patient "If you prefer, I will not write down your answers."

- Sometimes also reminding patients that these are routine medical questions asked of most patients will help them discuss something which may be difficult.
- Appropriate places to present a transitional statement are before the past medical and family histories; before the personal social history, i.e., questions about substance abuse including tobacco and alcohol, sexual history, intimate partner violence, and—in some cultures—menses; before the physical exam; moving from one region to another; and closing.

- **Before the past medical history:**

  "Okay, Mr. Green, now I'm going to ask you some questions about your health in general."

- **Before the sexual history:**

  "I am now going to ask you some personal questions regarding your sexual history. The answers will help me determine the reasons for your symptoms. Everything we discuss today will be kept confidential."

- **Before the social history:**

  "Thank you. Now let me ask you about your work and home life."

- **Before asking questions about smoking, alcohol, and recreational drug use:**

  "Okay, now I need to get some information about your habits and lifestyle."

- **Before the family history:**

  "Now let's talk about your family's health."

- **Before the physical exam:**

  "Thanks for answering all these questions. Now I'll need to examine you. Excuse me while I first wash my hands."

- **Before the closing:**

  "Thank you, Mrs. Jones. I have finished with my examination. I'd like to now sit down and discuss what I think so far."

> Without transitions, questions can be abrupt and confusing. Patients prefer to know what is happening next. Keep your SP informed and on track by using transitions.

28. Summarized significant information

Recent studies have shown that there is a strong positive relationship between the time spent doing the closure and the outcome on the CIS component of the CS exam. Therefore, be sure to give yourself enough time at the end of each encounter to complete your closure. This is your opportunity to pull everything together.

Before sharing your diagnostic impression, summarize 4 to 5 important points from the history and physical exam which have led to your preliminary conclusions. These points may be either pertinent positives or pertinent negatives. Remember this is part of your communication score and if you do not report the information accurately it will reflect negatively on your listening skills.

In order to use the limited amount of time provided for each encounter most efficiently, summarize only after completing both your history and physical examination. There is no need to stop and summarize at the completion of the history and then again after completing the physical examination. Your summary will be more complete and informative once all data gathering has been completed.

29. Delivered diagnostic impression

Next you need to state your diagnostic impression to the patient. First give the diagnosis in medical terms and then explain what the diagnosis means. Here, medical terminology should be used combined with an appropriate explanation.

- "I think you most likely have an ectopic pregnancy, which is a pregnancy growing outside of your womb."

Including the actual disease name shows respect for the intellectual capacity of the patient. Also, patients will feel comforted knowing that after the visit they have the ability to investigate on their own and learn more about their possible diagnosis. Once again, information can be comforting to patients. It is better to explain one disease properly than to list other possibilities in an unexplained fashion.

Many times the diagnosis you suspect is the most likely diagnosis for the case is one that is much less serious and more easily resolved than the one told to you by the patient when asked what the patient thinks is the cause of the chief complaint. If so, remember to inform the patient that you do not think they have the concerning disease. If the suspected diagnosis is more severe than suspected by the patient, you must frame the conversation differently and be prepared for a stronger reaction by the patient to the diagnosis.

When explaining the diagnosis to patients, consider referring to an organ or body system (heart, lungs, liver, immune system) and then state the general condition of that organ or system (infection, virus, blockage, inflammation). Remember that this is not a definitive but rather a possible diagnosis.

> When delivering the diagnosis, watch the SP carefully. If you have not yet pursued hidden concerns (item 22), this may be the moment when the SP will react based on his fears and concerns. If you missed this clue, the SP knows you were not focused on him.

30. Justified diagnosis

The SPs are well trained to play these cases and are quite knowledgeable about the mimicked diseases. Therefore, your choice of supporting facts from both the history and physical exam must accurately justify the given probable diagnosis. Also remember that you are being graded on your communications skills, where *how* you say something is relatively more important than what you say. Even if the diagnosis you select is not the most likely diagnosis for the case, but rather an appropriate differential diagnosis, you will still receive credit if it is explained properly and can be justified using the facts of the case.

31. Addressed patient's need for additional information

Illness will always be frightening to patients. Most often they will assume the worst possible cause of their symptoms. One thing that you as their physician can do to alleviate their fear is to help them understand what is happening. By providing patients with sufficient medical information in an understandable format you can put them at ease. Remember that you are trying to *decrease* uncertainty, not increase it, in your patients.

Carefully observe the patient's response to the diagnosis and later on to the proposed required tests. If the patient looks puzzled or says something like "Why do you think that is what is causing my CC or that this test will help confirm what is wrong?" remember to explain in further detail. The amount of information required by different patients may depend on their personality, level of education or level of distraction by the seriousness of the CC.

> If you acknowledge the SP's reaction to the diagnosis, it will lead you to determine whether he will want additional information. Focus on the SP and he will guide you.

32. Encouraged and answered questions

Always encourage the patient to ask questions—it is better to state, "What questions do you have?" instead of "Do you have any questions?" because the latter can be answered with yes/no. Then answer briefly in a clear and reassuring manner. Typically the SP should ask only the number of questions that can reasonably be answered in the available time. If you are asked more than you are capable of answering in the allotted time, reassure the patient that you will address all concerns at the follow-up visit.

- "I wish I had more time today to answer all your questions and address all your concerns. We can begin our next visit discussing the other issues you mentioned today."

> You have been asking the SP a number of questions for 14 minutes, and now he may want to ask one of you. Ask if he has any questions.

33. Assessed patient's comprehension of probable illness

Once you have provided the patient with all the information you deem necessary to understand the diagnosis, you must confirm with the patient that you have succeeded in achieving this goal. Ask if anything else needs to be clarified. By the time you leave the examining room, the patient should feel adequately informed, supported, and ready to take the next step.

> When the SP is informed and understands his situation, he will feel empowered.

34. Clearly stated next steps

By the end of the encounter, the patient should know what to do next. In most cases, this is accomplished by your stating which tests are necessary. Technical terminology should not be used in specifying lab work; however, it is imperative that you explain the purpose of the test. Never just say that we need to do further investigations with a vague reference to a test.

- "I will order a blood test to see if you have an infection."
- **NOT** "I will order a blood test" (too vague) or "I will order a CBC" (too technical)

This section also presents an additional opportunity to thank patients for sharing all the previously given information and letting them know that the information has helped in selecting the most appropriate tests to clarify their symptoms and confirm the correct diagnosis.

> Patients like to know what to do next. After informing the SP of the tests required, tell her what to do next, such as get dressed or relax in her seat until the nurse or technician comes.

35. Counseled the patient

It is very difficult to get patients to change their habits and lifestyle and to commit to following medical recommendations. It often helps for them to have family and/or friends who would be willing to assist. Therefore, try to identify the support network of your patients prior to introducing counseling. Then one thing you can suggest might be to have the patient involve one of those individuals in the process. Include any support available in the hospital or community, such as counseling or peer support groups for diabetes, lupus, cancer, etc. and social services for any financial concerns. Your goal should be to build a supportive therapeutic relationship with your patient.

Also, patients will more likely comply with your recommendations if they understand why they should do them. Raising their anxiety level a bit without overly alarming them can be effective.

- "As your physician I want you be as healthy as possible, so I am sending you to our counselor at the hospital who can help you cut down on the number of cigarettes you are smoking each day," **ADDING** "since cigarettes can harm your heart and lungs."

Another key point is to present counseling information to patients with empathic understanding about their clinical status. For example, a patient with severe recurrent hemoptysis and a history of cigarette smoking should be provided with plans for the management of the acute problem. Cigarette smoking can be addressed when the patient has improved.

- "A chest x-ray is needed, which I will review immediately. If you wish, I will provide you with information to help you stop smoking. It may be playing a role here, but let's first take care of this immediate problem."

Patients can be counseled about issues related to their general health and disease prevention, such as going for routine medical visits and age appropriate screening tests, diet, exercise, safe sex, cigarette and alcohol cessation and compliance with prescription medications. Occasionally, counseling can be more specific and related directly to the CC such as not driving with a seizure disorder.

You will be given credit for verbal counseling. USMLE guidelines clearly state, however, that counseling should be omitted from the Note. It is not considered part of the diagnostic plan.

> SPs feel 'taken care of' and confident when you counsel them in a non-judgmental manner. They know you are concerned about their health and best interest; when you treat them as a partner, it will make them more open and compliant with the proposed treatment.

36. Agreed to a mutual plan of action

During the encounter, you as the physician will advise the patient of the necessity to make lifestyle changes which will improve health and well-being. In addition, you will specify the tests needed to definitively diagnose the cause of the presenting complaint. To achieve these goals, the patient must agree to comply with all of your recommendations.

The patient needs to realize that you will always be available to help with this process. Make statements that are suggestive of a plan of action based on mutual involvement. Shared decision-making that includes the participation of the patient will create solutions that best fit the needs and personality of the individual patient.

- "We are a team."
- "We will figure this out together."
- "Let's work on this together."

- "How does this sound to you?"
- "Do you agree with this plan of action?"

It is imperative to uncover any barriers that could potentially interfere with achieving your stated goals. The patient must have both the motivation and capability to succeed. If a patient is not ready to agree to all your medical suggestions, the proposed and accepted mutual plan of action may be simply for the patient to agree to come for a follow-up visit and continue the discussion.

37. Actively listened and validated patient's experience

The final step in the process of showing empathy involves validating the patient's emotions. You may not agree with the emotion but you accept it without judgment and respect his right to feel that way. Be sure that patients feel legitimized and leave thinking that you accept them wholeheartedly with both their strengths and weaknesses.

- "Many of my patients with similar problems have felt the way you do."
- "I can understand why you would be worried under these circumstances. It would be surprising if you were not worried."
- "I can image that I would feel as you do if I had been through that."

38. Expressed empathy with appropriate reassurances

Empathy shows that you accurately understand what the patient is feeling and why they are feeling as they do. It starts with demonstrating to the patient that you understand, yet as the physician you are maintaining a level of emotional detachment. Every case should begin and end with an expression of empathy, with additional expression and non-verbal displays of empathy at appropriate times.

There are several types of situations that will give you the opportunity to prove your capacity to express empathy, and therefore be given exam credit for verbal expression of empathy.

- Patients describe emotions they are currently feeling, whether very positive or very negative about something physical or psychosocial
- Patients are open and tell you directly their concerns and how feeling this way has impacted their lives
- Patients simply state how they feel and need you to probe for additional details ("What do you think brought this on?" or "Tell me how this has affected you?")
- Patients simply state how they feel such as "my stomach really hurts," "I am so tired all the time" or "lately I don't seem to be able to concentrate on my job."
  - In these cases, acknowledge the statement and then ask about concerns connected to that statement. One patient with abdominal pain may fear she has cancer, another may be worried about the possible need for surgery, and yet another may worry that if it is something contagious she will not have anyone to take care of her children. You must determine the implications of that complaint to your individual patient.

Besides asking about the patient's concerns, as an alternative approach you can suggest how you think this problem has affected the patient. Do not merely acknowledge the complaint but explain what you think having the chief complaint means to the patient and how it may have affected them. If a patient presents with severe knee pain, show that it is important to you to understand the effect the pain has had on the patient's quality of life.

- "I can see you are in a lot of pain" ADDING "It must be difficult for you to walk around and perform many of your daily tasks."

Either way, by inviting further discussion on the subject and giving patients a chance to elaborate further, you are showing them that you are both listening and want to truly understand their feelings. Your patient should feel listened to as well as understood. Avoid statements such as "I know how you feel" or "I know what you are going through" because that may be considered presumptuous, trite, robotic, generic or insincere. You never want the patient to feel that you shifted the focus from them to you.

The final step in this process of showing empathy involves receiving confirmation from patients that you as the physician truly understood what they were feeling and why they feel that way. That confirmation will come in statements such as "Thank you for listening. That is exactly how I feel." or "Wow. You really understand how I am feeling." or simply "Yep. You got it."

The second type of situation that will give you an opportunity to express empathy will be more observational in nature. Learn to notice and interpret the non-verbal cues of patients who are anxious, sad, or angry.

- Patients are sitting with shoulders slumped, a sad facial expression, sighing and holding their bodies tensely, or breaking eye contact
  - In these cases, comment on what you notice and ask if there is something the patient would like to share verbally with you connected to their non-verbal communication. Even silence on the part of the patient may indicate that he or she is feeling something deeply and may be having trouble controlling his or her emotions.
  - On your part, empathic expression also involves non-verbal communication. Verbal and nonverbal communication should complement each other. Empathy can be communicated through facial expressions, appropriate body posture, mannerisms, and tone of voice. Changing your tone of voice can change the entire meaning of your words and can be used to acknowledge the patient's feelings and to show a genuine desire to help.

Sometimes a simple gesture like an appropriate placement of a hand on a patient's shoulder communicates warmth, caring and support. Assisting a patient to lie down or sit up by holding an arm or back demonstrates that you understand that it may be difficult to do so without help. Even a simple nod, or leaning in to listen, conveys to the patient that you are listening, absorbing information, and trying to understand.

Finally, while performing the PE, exhibiting appropriate caution can convey to patients an understanding of their current circumstances. Always examine the asymptomatic areas prior to the symptomatic ones. Warn the patient in advance prior to doing something unexpected or painful. If the patient appears to be in significant pain, when inquiring about the hospital gown, remembering to verbalize that you recognize that any shifting of position required to move the gown may exacerbate the pain, once again conveys understanding.

Be attentive to patient discomfort and do not cause any unnecessary pain by performing any maneuvers that yield no new data. If you suspect appendicitis and the psoas test is positive, do not perform an obturator test. Similarly, do not ask the patient to change positions more often than necessary, and thus causing any unecessary pain. (This could happen if, to complete your evaluation, you wanted to return to an area previously examined and thus asked a patient in pain to change position once again.)

The best way to communicate that you truly understand will be with appropriate reassurance. Be sure that your reassurances are consistent with the expectations and concerns of the patient.

- It is inappropriate to assure patients that they will get well or be cured, or to say that the condition isn't serious and not to worry if it is not. Reassure them instead that you will be extremely thorough and will help them get through this difficult time.

- Emphasize to patients that they are in a safe, modern medical center with an excellent medical staff.
- Offer your personal support and let patients know they are not alone.

Do not provide false reassurances with statements such as, "Don't worry, everything is going to be fine." Trust will not develop if the discussion is dishonest. If the patient is worried about something, she should be encouraged to speak further. Otherwise patients may think you do not take their feelings seriously.

It is important that you find empathic phrases which feel natural to you.

- That sounds very frustrating.
- This must be very frustrating for you.
- I notice that you seem to be feeling xxx.
- I want to understand what happened.
- I want to understand your feelings.
- What you seem to be saying is…is that correct?
- Can I help you put your feelings in words.
- Some people feel…. how do you feel?
- Am I hearing you right?
- It must be very difficult for you to cope with this.
- I recognize that this is a difficult time for you.
- I can understand how that could be upsetting.
- It sounds like you have been through a lot lately. I can understand how you would be upset.
- Let me make sure I understand your concerns.
- You seem angry, sad etc.
- You seem to be having trouble telling me about….
- It must be terrible feeling tired all the time where everything takes so much effort. Tell me how it affects you.
- What do you think might be going on?
- What do you think brought this on?
- How does that affect you?
- What do you fear most about this?

> Observe the SP and then acknowledge what you see in a sincere non-robotic way. Don't say you "know how he feels" since you may never have had the same experience. Acknowledge what you see—the mental, emotional, or physical state—and then offer reassurance that you are here for support.

39. Inquired about patient's support system

Patients will require help and support to deal with both acute and chronic problems. Support can include family, friends, work colleagues, clergy, therapists, support groups, and financial counselors. The form of support needed will depend on the situation. A patient who has to remain in the hospital may need emotional support as well as help with home and work obligations that cannot be fulfilled during the hospitalization. A person who needs to introduce lifestyle modifications such as an exercise regimen or a new diet may need a companion who has sufficient time available to eat and exercise with the patient.

Begin by asking the patient who in his life is available for support, and then offer additional and alternative support as needed. Most importantly, be sure that the patient knows you are always available to help in any way you can. Your recognition of the difficulty of achieving certain goals without appropriate support, as well as your commitment to help, reinforces the partnership you have created with the patient during the encounter.

40. Managed the challenge

Most challenges are testing one of several possible things. The first may be your ability to recognize an emotion the patient is displaying and why they may be feeling that way. If you encounter an angry patient, try to figure out why he is angry. He may state that he is angry because you made him wait so long to see you, but his anger might be indicative of something deeper and more complicated. In other words, his anger may be displaced; perhaps he is afraid of something such as being seriously ill for this first time or of losing control in a medical setting. Accept the fact that the patient is angry and do not get angry in return. Maintain your level of professionalism and composure and never become defensive.

Other challenges will be created to see if you, as a physician, are secure enough to admit further information is needed before you can commit to a diagnosis or treatment. Examples may be challenges from patients asking "Do I have cancer?" or "Am I going to die?" Be sure to explore why the patient has these concerns, express empathy, but do not feel obligated to answer these types of questions directly at this point in time. Reassure the patient that he is in good hands and that you will answer these questions when more information becomes available. The patient should understand exactly what you know/do not know and can/cannot do at this point in time. This approach creates a sense of trust.

Still others will really be a test of your information-sharing skills. Those may fall under the category of uncertainty because of something the patient does not understand. They will require you to provide the patient with appropriate medical information to minimize uncertainty and then with appropriate reassurances. For example, a patient may say "An ulcer. Oh no. My uncle died from an ulcer." Your response should be to obtain some more details and then explain to the patient how specific management of an ulcer can change the ultimate outcome, while reassuring the patient that this is a good hospital and you will personally manage the care. You are correcting the erroneous belief that everyone with an ulcer dies.

> SPs will always present you with a challenge, but they will not trick you. Everything they do is for a reason, so don't ignore it; just follow their lead.

CHALLENGING SCENARIOS

Patient with severe pain

Acknowledge the patients' pain and explain that you will give medication for it after you have evaluated the cause. Explain that you must first identify the cause in order to give the patient the best medication for the pain. For the pain of an acute abdomen, explain there will be a short delay in providing treatment until you have determined what medication is both needed and safe to be given. Help the patient get into the most comfortable position and save the examination of the painful region for last. Compassionately explain why an exam of this region is of importance; then perform the exam gently and quickly.

Patient who wants treatment without an exam

Mr. Thomas: "I really can't come in to see you. I have no health insurance—can't you just refill my pills? It's only $4 for a month's supply at Wal-Mart. If I do everything you say it will be a hundred times or a thousand times more!"

First, explain to the patient that you understand the current circumstances that have made it difficult to come to see you today. But then stress that there exists the necessity to periodically see patients with chronic medical disorders to review medications and evaluate for complications of the disease.

"I need to see you because you may need different or more medicine. I'll keep your concerns about cost in mind, however I'm going to recommend what is best for your health. I can have you speak with our counselor [social worker], who might be able to help you get health insurance."

Be sure not to promise that the counselor will be able to get the patient health insurance. Have the patient talk to the social worker, if only to see if she can help.

Ms. Gold: "I have a sore throat. My daughter had one a few days ago and her pediatrician gave her antibiotics. I am late for work, so please just give me some antibiotics so I can leave."

Use reassurance and compassion to explain why sometimes an antibiotic can be more harmful than helpful and therefore you want to be sure she needs antibiotics. Explain that doing an examination and performing needed tests is an excellent way to determine if she actually needs them and if so which ones.

Patient who asks if she has cancer

"I know this must be frightening, Mrs. Cheng. I want to understand why you think that you may have cancer. There are many problems other than cancer that can cause you to feel this way. I'll complete my exam, order tests, and have you return in a day or two to present my results with the reason for your symptoms. If it turns out to be something serious I will be there to help you and I have treatments we can try together."

Patient who asks if he is going to die

If asked this question in a case of breaking bad news, such as cancer, respond with honesty and hope–the two "Hs." Be honest about the prognosis and instill realistic hope. Let the patient know of the need to obtain the results of additional tests and to first try some form of treatment and assess the results in order to determine the actual prognosis. Emphasize the outstanding medical and nursing staff with the enormous modern resources available in "this medical center." The doctor is scored on his ability to be honest, reassuring, and empathic. It's a combination of what is said and how it is presented.

Patient who wants more information about a test

Describe tests in lay terms and with honesty, presenting information about discomfort or pain. Emphasize how tests help doctors to solve a patient's problem.

Angry patient

A patient may be angry because of a long wait or because other clinicians have been unable to solve his problem. Be prepared to manage these clinical challenges by identifying and discussing them with the patient. Validate the emotions the patient is feeling.

"Ms. White, I can see you are angry. I am sorry that I kept you waiting. I am here now and you have my complete attention." It is usually better not to offer a detailed explanation, such as "The reason that I was late and kept you waiting was that I had to see a patient in the emergency room." These types of explanation often create more rather than less resentment on the part of the patient.

Verbose patient

Redirecting the verbose patient to the essence of the history requires patience and finesse. At the right moment, gently interrupt and guide the patient back to a discussion of symptoms. Closed-ended questions are a great way to refocus the discussion.

Reluctant patient

How will a patient present with an unclear agenda? One example is the appointment which was made by another person without clarification about the reason for concern, e.g., an adolescent whose mother made the appointment for a "checkup." When faced with this challenge, begin with an open-ended question.

"Why is your mother concerned?"
"Now that you are here, how can I help you?"

"I would really like to help you. If you give me more details about your problem I can help you feel better."

The clinician needs to be patient and kind. If the patient persists in withholding important medical information, consider reassuring about confidentiality.

Patient who asks about HIV or AIDS as a reason for symptoms

Honesty is the key. If you believe it is a remote possibility that the patient is HIV-positive or has AIDS, explain that she is in a low-risk group and this is unlikely to explain the symptoms. If the patient is in a high-risk group with more typical symptoms, be more circumspect, stating the virus may be present but only testing will confirm it. Add that AIDS is now managed as a chronic condition similar to diabetes or hypertension.

Patient with decreased vision or hearing

If a patient has poor vision, tell her where in the room you are sitting and help her with any maneuvers she may need to perform. If the patient has decreased hearing, sit close and speak into the stronger ear.

Patient with intimate partner violence (IPV)

Intimate partner violence is defined as actual or threatened physical, sexual, psychological, and emotional abuse by a current or former partner. IPV is a major challenge because those being abused are ashamed and reluctant to share this information, even with a physician. Patients who experience IPV often present with a somatic symptom that has not been linked to IPV by other physicians. A subtle hint may be if she looks away or becomes teary-eyed when asked about her home or family. Use the SAFE acronym; ask, "Is she concerned about her Safety or the Safety of her children; does she feel Afraid; does she have supportive Friends and/or Family; and, has she made an Emergency plan?" Reassure the patient that you are there to help, by offering medical center resources and support to her and her partner. Remind her that everything is confidential.

Patient who requests that you lie on a form

> Mr. Brown: "Doc, could you just put down on the form that everything is normal? I really need this insurance."

Mr. Brown has just requested that you lie. Apart from not committing insurance fraud, the key to this challenge is to stay calm, non-defensive, and nonjudgmental. Reply with a statement such as, "I'm afraid I can't do that. For now, let us work together to make your health better." If the patient is insistent about what he believes you should include in the form, simply give him back the blank form.

> Mr. Davis: "Please give me the note that states that I am in good health for the job of taxi driver and I'll be on my way. Also Doc, just to let you know, I have the cash on me to pay you."

Apart from not providing the note, the key here is to remain non-defensive and nonjudgmental about the fact that an attempt was just made to bribe you. Just smile, and do what is in the patient's best interest. Be honest and state clearly "I cannot write that note today. I am concerned about your drinking and the falls you have had. I believe you may put yourself and others at risk if you drive a taxi in your current state of health. I would like you to see our alcohol counselor, and we will meet soon after you have the picture of your head. In fact, I'd like to arrange to take the picture now."

PRACTICE CASE

The case that follows gives you the opportunity to test your level of understanding of the 40 skills above and shows you examples of how to appropriately incorporate each one of them into any individual case.

Cover the right side of the page and see if you can identify examples of each one of the communication skills from the checklist. If you cannot, review the checklist and explanations and then try again.

PRACTICE CASE: SEVERE ABDOMINAL PAIN

Doorway Information

Opening Scenario

Susan Albright is a 35-year-old woman who comes to the ER complaining of severe abdominal pain.

Vital Signs

T 37.0 C (98.6 F), BP 120/78 mm Hg, HR 100/min (regular), RR 19/min

Pulse oximetry 92% on room air

Examinee Tasks

1. Obtain a focused history.

2. Perform a relevant physical exam. Do not perform rectal, pelvic, genitourinary, female breast, or corneal reflex exam.

3. Discuss your initial diagnostic impression and your workup plan with the patient.

4. After leaving the room, complete your Patient Note.

CIS Skill	Sample Doctor–Patient Interaction
1. Knocked	Knock, Knock, Knock

Patient: Come in

5. Professional appearance

Enter the room wearing a clean white lab coat over professional attire. Notice that the patient is lying on the table in a fetal position facing the right side. When you enter the room her back is to you. She is already draped to the waist. Walk around the table to face the patient.

2. Introduced self
4. Clarified role
3. Patient's preferred title

Doctor: Hello Ms. Albright? My name is Dr. Levine. I am a doctor at this hospital and will be taking care of you today. I will be asking you questions, examining you and taking a few notes to be sure I have a record of all the important information. How would you like to be addressed?

Patient: Please call me Ms. Albright.

9. Attention and concentration

Doctor: Ok. Ms. Albright, you look uncomfortable on the examination table. Let me pull out the leg rest so you will be more comfortable while we speak. I will try to be efficient in obtaining all the important information so we can determine what is causing your pain and the best way to treat it.

11. Eye contact
12. Distance
15. Elicited chief complaint

Sit down on the patient's right side at a 45-degree angle and approximately 2-3 feet away.

Doctor: What caused you to come see me today?

Patient: I am having really terrible stomach pain.

Doctor: Please point to the pain

Patient points to right lower quadrant

Doctor: Thank you. On a scale of 1 to 10, where 10 is the worst pain you have ever had, and 1 is a mild pain, how would you rate this pain?

Patient: It is terrible. I would call it a 10 out of 10.

38. Empathy and reassurance

Doctor: I can see you are in a lot of pain. It must have been very difficult for you to even walk into the hospital to come see me today.

Patient: Yes, it was. Thank you for noticing and caring.

17. Open-ended question

Doctor: How would you describe your pain? (What does the pain feel like to you?)

Patient: It feels sharp, almost like someone is taking a knife and stabbing me on my side.

16. Timeline of CC

Doctor: When did it start?

Patient: About 6 hours ago

Doctor: Did it come on suddenly or more gradually?

Patient: Very suddenly

Doctor: Is it there all the time, or does it come and go?

Patient: It is there all the time.

Doctor: Is it staying the same or getting better or worse?

Patient: Worse

Doctor: What were you doing when the pain first started? (Can you think of anything that might have brought it on?)

Patient: Nothing in particular. I was just sitting and watching television and all of a sudden it hit me.

Doctor: Does it move anywhere?

Patient: No

Doctor: Did it start where it is now?

Patient: Yes

Doctor: So the pain has always been on your lower right side.

Patient: Yes it has.

Doctor: Ok, so does anything make it worse?

Patient: If I move or take a deep breath it gets worse.

Doctor: Have you tried anything to make it better?

Patient: I took some Advil I have at home and use once in a while. I thought I would feel fine after that.

Doctor: Did it work at all?

Patient: No

Doctor: Besides the pain, have you been nauseous?

Patient: Yes. A little.

Doctor: Did you vomit?

Patient: No

Doctor: So you feel nauseous, but did not vomit. Is that correct?

Patient: Exactly

Doctor: Do you have diarrhea?

Patient: No

Doctor: Have you had a fever?

Patient: I did not take my temperature, but I do not feel warm.

Doctor: How has your appetite been?

Patient: I have not eaten today because the pain is so bad, but I do feel a little bit hungry.

Doctor: Any burning when you urinate?

Patient: No

Doctor: Have you noticed any discharge or liquid coming out of your vagina?

Patient: No

Annotations
17. Open-ended question
21. Paraphrased
17. Open-ended question
18. Closed-ended question
18. Closed-ended question
21. Paraphrased
19. Non-leading question

19. Non-leading question

Doctor: Any spotting?

Patient: Yes. When I went to the bathroom before, I noticed a little blood on the tissue.

Doctor: Ok. So when was your last menstrual period?

P: Now that I think about it, I am a little late. It was about 6 weeks ago.

D: Are your periods regular?

P: Yes. Very. I get my period every 28 days.

D: Have you noticed any other symptoms since the pain started?

P: No

27. Transitional phrase

D: Now I am going to ask you some questions about your past health.

P: Okay

D: Have you ever had pain like this before?

P: Never

D: Are you allergic to or have had a strange reaction to any medication?

P: No

D: Are you taking any medication prescribed for you by a physician?

P: No

D: How about anything you may have bought over the counter without a prescription, besides the Advil you mentioned?

P: No

D: Have you ever been hospitalized?

P: Yes, when I was 14 I had surgery for my appendix that burst. And it happened when my parents were away and I was staying at a friend's house.

14. Non-verbal ease

Lean in and nod

38. Empathy and
    reassurance

D: Sounds like you were pretty sick. Being in a hospital and having surgery in itself would be frightening for a 14 year old. But being alone until your parents could get there must have made it even more difficult for you.

P: Yes it was. Until my parents arrived I felt lonely and scared. And then I was in pain for a while and missed 2 weeks of school.

D: I can understand how upset you must have been

P: Yes I was

D: Have you had any accidents or injuries, especially in the stomach area where you have your pain?

P: No

D: Do you have any medical problems?

P: I once had a urine infection but that is about it. I had some pain then but this feels different.

D: Have you ever had any other surgery besides having your appendix removed?

P: No

D: Recently have you noticed any changes in your urination?

P: No

D: Any blood in your urine?

P: No

D: Any changes in your bowel movements?

P: No

D: Any changes in the size of your stomach area?

P: No

D: Any changes in your weight?

P: No

D: Have you recently traveled?

P: No

D: Does anyone in your family have the same pain you have?

P: As far as I know, I am the only one who is sick.

D: Any serious illnesses run in your family?

P: Uh. Let me see.

Give patient time to think and do not proceed yet with the next question.

P: No

D: Have you ever been pregnant?

P: No

D: I am now going to ask you some questions about your sexual history, which is a routine part of the history when a woman has lower abdominal pain. I want you to remember that everything you tell me is confidential. Are you currently sexually active?

P: Yes I am.

D: How many partners do you have now?

P: Right now just my boyfriend.

D: How many in the past?

P: During the last 10 years, I would say about 20.

D: Do you use condoms?

P: Yes

19. Non-leading question

20. Clear and concise questions, one at a time

19. Non-leading question

10. Did not interrupt

27. Transitional phrase
16. Non-leading question

D: Do you use them consistently?

P: We try to, but we forget many times.

8. Non judgmental

D: Thank you.

25. Lay language

D: Do you use any other form of birth control?

P: No

25. Lay language

D: Have you ever had an infection that was transmitted sexually?

P: Yes. Last year I went to my doctor because I had stomach pain,

26. Use of continuer

D: Uh-huh

P: A fever, and a discharge and was told I had PID.

D: Have you ever been tested for HIV, the AIDS virus?

P: I have not.

27. Transitional phrase
19. Non-leading question

D: I am now going to ask you some questions about your habits. Have you ever used tobacco in any form?

P: No

D: Do you drink alcohol?

P: Just socially

10. Repeated question for clarification

D: I want to try and better understand how much alcohol you drink. Can you explain what you mean by drinking alcohol socially?

P: My boyfriend and I have an occasional glass of wine with dinner.

D: Have you ever used recreational drugs?

P: Never. I think drugs are dangerous.

D: Is there anything else about your health that you would like to tell me that I have not asked?

P: No. I think I have told you everything.

27. Transitional phrase

D: Thank you for answering my questions. Now I need to examine you. Before I begin, excuse me while I wash my hands.

6. Care and concern

Wash your hands. (If using hand sanitizer, remember to let the SP see you rubbing your hands together.)

38. Empathy and reassurance

Remember to begin the physical exam in the patient's current position. Do not ask a patient in pain to move more than is necessary.

8. Respect

D: I know you can't see what I am doing so I will explain everything to you.

P: Thank you.

13. Draping
38. Empathy and reassurance

D: While I examine you, your gown will need to be untied, retied, raised and lowered. Can I help you by doing these things for you?

P: It would be easier if you did it for me. Thank you for offering.

Untie and raise the gown.

D: I need to tap on your back.

Check for CVAT, costovertebral angle tenderness, on the right and left sides.

Lower gown and retie it.

D: I know you are in a lot of pain, but I need to check a few more things that will help me figure out what is wrong. To do this I need you to turn on your back. If it is difficult for you to do this, I can help you turn.

P: Thank you for offering but I can do it myself.

Hold the drape while the patient turns on her back.

D: I am going to take a look at your stomach area.

As agreed upon at the beginning of the physical exam, raise the gown after lowering the drape.

Inspect the abdomen.

D: I need to listen to your stomach.

Auscultate the abdomen in 4 quadrants. Order – RUQ, LUQ, LLQ, RLQ

D: I need to tap on your stomach. Let me know if this causes more pain.

Percuss all 4 quadrants in the same order.

D: I need to press on your stomach. It may hurt but I will be as gentle and quick as possible.

Palpate all 4 quadrants, going last to the RLQ.

P: That really did hurt on my right side.

D: I am so sorry that caused you pain but it gave me some very important information.

I need to press deeper, but I will only press in the areas that did not hurt you. I will not press on your right side again.

P: Thank you.

Palpate deeply the other 3 quadrants.

D: I am going to press on your lower left side. Let me know if it hurts more when I press or when I let go.

P: When you let go.

D: Thank you for allowing me to examine your belly. I know that part of this examination was uncomfortable.

Lower the gown and recover the patient with the drape.

D: Do you want to stay in this position or turn again on your side while I tell you what I am thinking? I want you to be as comfortable as possible while I explain everything to you.

P: I am in a lot of pain and prefer not to move again.

D: First, to summarize, you told me you have had severe pain on your lower right side for 6 hours, that you have had a small amount of vaginal spotting, that your last menstrual period was 6 weeks ago, and that you have had PID in the past. When I pressed on your right lower side it was extremely painful for you. Before I tell you what I am thinking

Margin annotations:
8. Respect
9. Attention and concentration
6. Care and concern
25. Lay language
7. Connected and purposeful PE
38. Empathy and reassurance
7. Connected and purposeful PE
13. Draping
38. Empathy and reassurance
6. Care and concern
28. Summarized
30. Justified diagnosis
24. What patient thought was going on

I would like to know what you think is causing your pain. The reason I am asking is that I want to be sure I address all your concerns, explain things properly with enough information, and correct any misinformation you may have.

P: A friend of mine had pain like this and her period was also late and she ended up with a pregnancy that ruptured in her abdomen.

29. Diagnostic impression
34. Summarized plan

D: I do think your problem also is most likely what we call an ectopic pregnancy, which is a pregnancy that is growing outside your womb. To be sure, I am going to order some tests. The first will be a blood test to check if you are pregnant. The second will be a picture of your stomach area to look for the pregnancy. I will get the results as soon as possible and let you know them.

P: From my friend I know a pregnancy outside my womb could be very serious and dangerous.

38. Empathy and Reassurance
37. Validated feelings

39. Support system

D: I understand your concerns. However, there is no need to be unnecessarily concerned at this time. The most important thing is that you are here now at this excellent hospital with very competent doctors. I want to reassure you that I will figure out what is wrong, and if it is serious, we will discuss together and agree on a treatment. I will do everything I can to help you get through this and be there for you until your problem is resolved.

Observe patient for reaction.

22. Hidden concern

D: You still look very worried to me. Is there something else that concerns you that you would be willing to share?

23. Impact on patient's life

P: Yes. I am afraid I may need surgery, and when I had my appendix removed I was very sick and it took a while to recover. Also, my sister is getting married in 2 weeks and I am her maid of honor.

37. Validated feelings

36. Mutual plan

35. Counseling

32. Asked if patient had questions

D: Of course that would be concerning to you. If you do end up needing surgery, it will likely be less invasive than your previous surgery. It can be done with a small incision and camera, and you will be home in a day or two and recover much quicker. For now let's take it together one step at a time. Also, I will talk to you in more detail when you are feeling better about using condoms/having safe sex until you are ready to get pregnant. I want to be sure you understand everything that is happening and everything that I have told you. What questions do you have for me?

P: None right now.

33. Assessed comprehension

D: Can I clarify anything I have told you?

P: I understand everything so far.

39. Support system

D: Is there anyone here with you or someone you would like us to call to come be with you?

36. Mutual plan

P: I was alone when I called the ambulance. So first let's get back my test results and depending what comes next I may call my boyfriend.

31. Assessed need for more Information

D: Is there anything else that is still concerning you right now?

P: No. Now that I understand what may be wrong and what will happen next I am less worried. But, can you give me something for pain?

40. Managed the challenge

D: I will make sure your test results are returned as quickly as possible. As soon as I know what is causing your pain and I am sure that it is safe, I will give you something for the pain.

P: Thank you.

D: Goodbye.

Spoken English Proficiency (SEP)

Spoken English Proficiency

3

Spoken English Proficiency (SEP) is about understandability in as far as it does not impair or hinder communication. It is not about your accent; it's about how well you and the Standardized Patient (SP) understand each other. The goal is verbally communicating in a way that strengthens the doctor-patient relationship.

COMPONENTS OF SEP GRADING

Five components comprise the grading of SEP:

1. **Pronunciation:** the effect that mispronounced words—not accents—limit comprehension of the questions or comments of the doctor. SPs are specifically trained to listen through accents.

2. **Word choice:** how the words and their component parts combine to form sentences. **Avoid using the same words repeatedly**. Vary your choice of words but keep it simple and use short sentences. The correct use of grammar is also taken into consideration, especially because incorrectly stating something as past when it is present, or present when it is past, because it can mislead the patient to (a) not be concerned, or (b) be overly concerned.

3. **Doctor's questions and responses being understood by the SP:** the patient does not need to ask the doctor to repeat questions or comments due to lack of understanding.

   If this happens repeatedly, it will affect your SEP score. Do not ignore the SP if he says, "I do not understand." Use different words to ask the same question. For example:

Doctor:	"Do you have angina?"
SP:	"What do you mean?"
Doctor:	"Do you have chest pain?"
SP:	"Oh, yes I do."

4. **SP's questions and responses being understood by the doctor:** the doctor does not need the SP to repeat responses or questions due to lack of understanding.

5. **Listener's effort:** the degree of listening effort that is necessary for the SP to understand the doctor. If you use simpler words, it will be less effort for the SP. Listener's effort can be affected by numerous things:
   - Talked too fast
   - Talked too slow
   - Talked too loud
   - Talked too soft
   - Mumbled

COMPONENTS OF SEP TIME-MANAGEMENT

Doctors are concerned about time management and the 15 minutes that have been allotted for each encounter. SPs are concerned about the time allotment as well.

- SPs have been trained to work within 15 minutes and will adjust their pace so as not to impede you from completing the task required.
- You do not need to speed up your dialogue since that may impair understandability, especially if you have an accent.
- Sometimes responding inappropriately to an SP's question can be interpreted as not understanding or not listening.
  - SPs may use idiomatic phrases or slang whose meaning you do not comprehend. If you are unsure, ask them what they mean.
  - It is not a mark against understandability if you ask for clarity. Do not pretend to understand the SP's meaning. Asking for clarity will strengthen your communication with your SP.
  - There is another skill you can demonstrate if you do not understand your SP. You can paraphrase (repeat back) in your own words what you believe was said. For example:

    SP: "I've been scratchy and hot for 3 days."

    Dr. "You've been scratching and had a fever for 3 days?"

    SP: "No, I've had a sore throat."

    Dr. "Okay, thank you."

Now you have paraphrased (giving you credit in communication skills) and clarified information to avoid misunderstanding and possible medical error.

RECOMMENDATIONS FOR IMPROVING SEP

If you practice speaking English every day, it will strengthen your confidence, giving you a comfort level which will surely help you to speak more freely with your SP during the encounters.

- Read out loud every day (the newspaper is a good source)
- Record your conversations and then evaluate them. Look to see if you do the following:
  - Mumble
  - Speak too fast or too slow
  - Speak too loud or too soft
  - Do not enunciate words sufficiently

Once you are aware of how you are perceived, record another conversation and notice the improvements.

- Focus and listen without considering your next question or response. This will help to decrease your misunderstandings and strengthen your ability to understand your SP. SEP is about understandability NOT your accent.
- Keep it simple. Use language that is easy to understand and avoid medical jargon.
- Vary your word choices and phrases.

"It is what you say but, more importantly, it's about **how** you say it."

Integrated Clinical Encounter (ICE)

Focused History-Taking

4

This section provides a list of suggested questions to be asked during patient history-taking. Not all of the questions are necessary or relevant to each patient encounter. It is your job, as the physician, to determine the appropriate historical questions to ask. Each question should be focused on the chief complaint, HPI, and aspects of the history related to the CC and HPI. Asking questions that are not relevant to the case will not earn you "more points"; it will only take time away from your ability to ask the appropriate questions.

While you are taking a good focused history from a patient, you need to **listen carefully**. You'll want to listen not only to the words you hear, but also to the tone. You'll also want to observe the patient's **body language**. Be astute in recognizing when the patient looks away, pauses, gets defensive, or becomes angry about a particular question you ask. These behaviors are there for a reason, and you have to be curious enough to dig a little deeper, always in a kind and reassuring manner.

THE MEDICAL INTERVIEW

During the Step 2 CS exam, the primary task is to generate differential diagnoses (hypotheses) with diagnostic and therapeutic plans. The Patient Note should clearly reflect this process, emphasizing primary data from the 15-minute patient encounter.

Introductory (Doorway) Information

Preliminary (introductory) information about the patient is available on the doorway of the examination room with additional copies inside the room and where you write the note. It provides name, age, gender, and the chief concern or complaint. Vital signs are listed:

- Temperature in degrees Fahrenheit and Centigrade (T)
- Blood pressure (BP)
- Heart rate (HR)
- Respiratory rate (RR)

Instructions are given on the tasks needed to complete during the encounter. Unless otherwise stated, it is implied that you will need to perform a physical examination on every SP. A case where a physical examination is not required is a telephone encounter. Read the instructions carefully and begin generating hypotheses that will lead to the correct diagnosis. Generating hypotheses helps save time by narrowing initial questioning to the most likely possibilities. Being a diligent listener will enable the addition or elimination of diagnoses.

PERFORMING THE FOCUSED HISTORY

Chief Complaint (CC)

This is usually a one-sentence description of the patient's reason for the visit.

- In actual practice in the United States, a nurse records this information given from the patient; the nurse writes it on the chart along with the patient's age and sex.
- The nurse then takes the vital signs. (You will accept all vitals signs as accurate.)
- The physician reviews this information prior to entering the room. At this point, the physician is already formulating a differential diagnosis, using only the age, sex, chief complaint and vital signs.
- The physician then enters the room and introduces himself. At this point, a focused history is performed.

An excellent way to start taking the history is to ask an open-ended question. This will give the patient an opportunity to "tell her story." For example:

> "Good morning/afternoon, Mrs. Santos. My name is Dr. Reina. I'm a doctor here in the hospital. I see you are here for chest pain. Can you tell me more about it?"

OR

> "Hello, Mr. Smith, I'm Dr. Wells. I will be taking care of you today. I see that you are here for an ankle injury. Can you tell me more about it?"

Listen closely and focus on what the patient is telling you. The anxiety on the day of the exam may be a strong distraction; however, with practice you will learn to master this skill.

You'll need to **avoid asking questions about something the patient has already stated**. For example, if the patient answers your open-ended question of "Can you tell me more about it?" with "Well, I hurt my ankle yesterday during a 5K race. I twisted it on the curb," and you then ask *when* it occurred, the patient will respond, "Yesterday." Now the patient knows that you have *not been listening*. Remember to listen to his story.

History of Present Illness

After you make your introduction, make the patient comfortable (*offering the drape/dimming the lights/adjusting the table*) and ask your open-ended question, obtain the **history of present illness (HPI)**. If the patient has already told you everything, you may move on to the PMH/ Meds/Allergies, etc. This may occur with a simple acute ankle injury.

Most patients, however, do not tell the whole story. They do not know what is important versus what is useless information. It is your job, as the physician, to elicit the important information.

This is the time when a mnemonic may help. Consider a mnemonic to be a road map that will keep you on the path of correct questions. Use it simply as a tool to help you obtain a complete, yet focused, HPI.

Using a mnemonic will help you overcome those stressful moments when you cannot think of any questions to ask. Jot it down on your scrap paper prior to entering the room. If you have memorized it well, simply shooting your eyes down to your notes momentarily to see the mnemonic will help trigger your memory, and help you to ask a question that you may otherwise have forgotten.

SIQOR A6

This mnemonic stands for the following:

    Site/Symptom

    Intensity/Quantity

    Quality

    Onset

    Radiation

    Aggravating Factors

    Alleviating Factors

    Associated Manifestations

    Attributions (what do you think caused this?)

    Adaptations (how does it affect your lifestyle?)

    Additional Concerns (hidden concerns)

Site

Patients generally refer to bodily location in lay terms and broadly rather than specifically, e.g., "headache," "stomachache," or "backache." The clinician must precisely identify the exact location; it is helpful to have the patient identify the area by pointing.

    "Please show me exactly where the pain is."

    "Can you point to where it hurts?"

Intensity/Quantity

Questions related to quantity include frequency, size, volume, and number. "How many times did you vomit today?" "How often does the stomach pain occur?" A patient may say that he's been coughing up "a lot of blood," when it turns out to be less than a teaspoon. The intensity of a symptom may be ascertained by asking the patient to use the 1 to 10 scale. The degree of functional impairment is quantified by getting specific details about what a patient can do and for how long.

    "If 10 is the worst pain you've ever had, where is this on a scale of 1 to 10?"

Quality

Begin by generally asking what the symptom feels like. If vague terms are used, ask the patient to relate it to a previous similar pain. It is often necessary for the clinician to ask specific questions:

    "How would you describe the pain (feeling, discomfort)?"

    "Please describe how it feels."

    "Tell me what it feels like."

If patient needs prompting:

    "Is it a dull ache (sharp, stabbing, burning, pulling, pulsating, cramping, pressure)?"

    "Does it come and go?"

    "Is the pain there all the time?"

Onset

Dates and times when symptoms first began are consistently the most reliable descriptors of the present illness. Ideally, the patient already gave you the chronology of events after your open-ended question in the beginning. If not, be sure to ask the patient about the very first time the symptom occurred. Patients may minimize early prodromal symptoms that seem unimportant to them but which are very critical diagnostically. Rapidly establish the last time a patient was in a normal state of health; ask one of these questions after inquiring about the chief complaint:

"When were you last in perfect health?"

"When did this first begin?" or "How long have you had this?"

"Have you ever had anything like this before?"

"Can I assume you were in perfect health prior to this?"

Establish the setting in which the patient's illness has developed and the location and time when symptoms occur; this adds precision to the HPI. "Setting" refers to where and when symptoms occur. The frenzy of an office at tax preparation time is obviously relevant when an accountant comes in with burning epigastric pain. For someone who has diarrhea, a recent trip abroad is relevant. Shortness of breath waking a patient in the early hours of the morning is a clue to the presence of congestive heart failure. Exertional chest pain is consistent with coronary artery disease.

"How often do you have this?"

"When do you get these pains (feelings)?"

"When does this occur? What time of day? What are you doing when the pain comes on?"

Radiation

"Questions related to radiation, i.e., movement, are helpful because patients often can tell, in a general way, whether pain or another symptom feels on the surface of their body or deep within."

"Does the pain (or other symptom) move anywhere? Show me where."
(Note: Don't use the word "radiate.")

"Do you feel the pain (or other symptom) anywhere else?"

"Does it ever travel to any other part of your body?"

"Does this pain ever move around?"

Patients are often under stress when they see the doctor, and misunderstandings are frequent. It is helpful to remember common patterns of pain radiation.

Type of Pain	Typically Radiates To
Ischemic chest pain	Arms, neck, back, mandible
Kidney stone	Femoral triangle and testes or vulva
Gallbladder	Posterior right shoulder region
Spleen injury, ruptured ectopic pregnancy	Top of the shoulders (diaphragm irritation)
Testicular torsion	Lower abdomen
Abdominal aortic aneurysm	Back, thoracic region
Pancreatitis	Back, thoracic region
Posterior penetrating gastric ulcer	Back, thoracic region
Lumbar disk herniation	Down lower limb, calf
Pharyngitis pain	Can radiate to ear

Aggravating factors

Questions that elucidate what conditions surround the onset of the symptoms are important. Questions that identify what worsens symptoms provide key information leading you to a more accurate differential diagnosis. Common factors include position, activity level, exertion, relation to food, time of day, and medication use.

"Are you aware of anything that might have brought this on?"

"What happened right before this came on (started)?"

"Did anything unusual happen at that time?"

"Does anything make your pain worse?"

"What makes it worse?"

Alleviating factors

Elucidate the reasons for symptom improvement; this provides additional information. Common factors: position, activity level, exertion, relation to food, time of day, and medication use.

"Does anything make your pain better?"

"What makes it better?"

Associated manifestations

Ask about other specific symptoms associated with the generated hypotheses, i.e., ask a young woman with joint pain about dermatitis and fever if systemic lupus erythematosus is a possible diagnosis.

Asking for "any other symptoms" will have a low yield because SPs are trained to respond with a vague answer: "What do you want to know, doctor?" Your question instead should be:

> "In addition to your headache, have you noticed anything else (e.g., nausea, vomiting, cough, fever, fatigue, loss of appetite, dizziness, cold, sore throat, weakness in your legs, tingling sensation, burning sensation, numbness, sweating)?"

Associated manifestations for cough are fever, sputum, dyspnea, chest pain, and hemoptysis. Associated manifestations for joint pain are redness, swelling, warmth, tenderness, and decreased range of motion

Adaptations

It can be valuable to ask how a patient's symptoms have affected his or her lifestyle. That can be helpful in determining the severity of a symptom. It can also potentially elucidate hidden concerns by the patient or other psychosocial factors. As this type of questioning can demonstrate your concern for the patient's quality of life, it will likely improve the personal rapport you are trying to establish. Your question should be:

> "How does this affect your lifestyle?" or "How does this affect you at work?" or "How does this affect you at home?"

Attribution

Oftentimes patients will have an idea what is causing their symptoms. This can either provide a clue to diagnosis or, if not medically accurate, reveal an area of concern for the patient. Perhaps a patient thinks he has cancer. If that is a diagnostic possibility, then that should be explored. If not, however, you can reassure the patient and alleviate his concern. Your question should be:

> "What do you think is causing your symptoms?"

Additional Concerns

Sometimes patients have additional concerns that have not been uncovered in other lines of questioning. Perhaps they are concerned that they will need to be hospitalized and that they will need to find someone to take care of their children. Other hidden concerns could include wanting pain medication, concerns about having cancer, needing surgery, death etc. Once you discover a concern, you should address it in an appropriate way. Your question should be:

> "What other concerns do you have?"

Other Components of the Patient's History

During the CS exam, the emphasis is on the HPI. Other aspects of the history are included if they are relevant to the HPI. Details of the present illness will guide one to the related components of the past medical history, family history, social history, and review of systems (symptoms). This flow of questioning allows you to test and refine your diagnostic hypotheses, and provide pertinent positive and negative information to include in the Patient Note.

Past Medical History

Past Medical History (PMH) is a relevant review of systems and symptoms, serious illnesses, hospitalizations, surgeries, medications, diets, weight changes, and sleep patterns.

One mnemonic is **PAMHRFOSS** (Ask relevant questions only):

- Previous event similar to the chief complaint
- Allergies (to foods, medicines, plants, animals)
- Medicines (OTC, prescriptions, vitamins, herbs)
- History of hospitalization/illnesses/trauma/surgery (HITS)
- Review of systems
- Family history (focused on problems similar to patient's CC and HPI)
- Ob/Gyn (e.g., last menstrual period [LMP], gravida, para, abortions, infections)
- Sexual history (sexually active, male/female/both, condom use or other method of contraception, STDs, number of partners in past 10 years, sexual function)
- Social history (occupation, home life, exercise, smoking, alcohol, illegal drugs)

Specific Phrases for PAMHRFOSS:

PAMHRFOSS: Previous episodes of chief complaint

"Have you ever had this before?"

You may already know the answer to this important question by asking about the symptom's frequency. If a patient has recurrent episodes of an identical headache, the diagnosis is more likely migraine or muscle contraction headache. If it's a new-onset headache in an elder, consider other diagnoses, such as cerebral vascular disease, subdural hematoma, neoplasm, or temporal arteritis.

PAMHRFOSS: Allergies

"Do you have any allergies?"

This is the basic question that must be asked to each patient. All patients need to be asked about allergies to medications. You also need to determine what the symptom is (patients are often confused and believe a side effect is in fact an allergy) to be sure it is an actual allergy. Diarrhea from antibiotics is not an allergy but patients may believe it is.

Patients may also have allergies to foods, plants, animals or environmental sources. If appropriate for the case, these issues may also need to be addressed. With a 25-year-old woman complaining of a cough for 6 months, for example, you might find out that she moved in with her boyfriend 6 months ago, and that her boyfriend has a cat. Upon further questioning, you find out that she experiences this same type of cough whenever she visits her grandmother (who also has a cat).

If an acute allergic reaction (rash, shortness of breath, anaphylaxis) is in your initial differential diagnosis, a more detailed allergy history is indicated. For example:

"Do you have any allergies to prescription medication?"

"How about any bad reaction to over-the-counter pills or herbal remedies?"

"Any reactions to food?"

"Have you ever had an allergy to shellfish or iodine?"

"Do you have any allergies to animals or plants?"

If you aren't sure you covered all the categories, you may also ask:

"Anything else you can tell me about allergies?"

PAMHRFOSS: Medications

Medications are extremely important. You'll need to ask about medications from each of your patients. There are 3 things to remember:

- Medication (name and why it was prescribed)
- When it was prescribed or stopped (Does that relate to the chief complaint?)
- Is the patient compliant with the medication?
- Is the patient experiencing any common side effects of the medication?

Medication history is inclusive of all of the following categories.

- Prescription medications
- Over-the-counter (OTC)
- Vitamin supplements or herbs
- Oral contraceptives

Some questions which may be important are the following:

"Are you taking any prescription medications?"

"Do you take anything over-the counter, like Tylenol® or aspirin?"

"Do you take oral birth control pills?"

"Do you take any vitamin supplements or herbs?"

"Are you experiencing any side effects from this medication? (If patient is taking a beta blocker, ask about depression and erectile dysfunction; if patient is taking an ACE inhibitor, ask about a dry cough; if patient is taking a calcium-channel blocker, ask about lower extremity swelling.)

For most cases you need only the **drug name**. Dose and frequency may be important if they relate to the chief complaint or your differential diagnosis. For example, a patient complaining of shortness of breath may have been told to take his Lasix® (furosemide) 2x a day. He chose to take it only 1x a day because he did not like getting up in the middle of the night to urinate. He is now in congestive heart failure because he was not compliant with his medications. One of the diagnoses you would list is, "*congestive heart failure due to non-compliance of diuretic.*"

If you are not familiar with a drug, ask **why it was prescribed** (this will be a natural lead-in to the past medical history which comes next) or **how it is spelled**.

PAMHRFOSS: History of Hospitalizations, etc.

The PMH will tell you a lot about the patient. A healthy patient who does not take any medications and sees his physician regularly is most likely a healthy patient. There is no need to ask about specific diseases.

The HITS can be divided into 4 components:

- Hospitalizations (**H**)
- Major illness (**I**)
- Significant trauma (**T**)
- Surgical history (**S**)

Hospitalizations

If a hospitalization was recent, new symptoms or complaints may be a complication or progression of the problem.

"Have you ever been hospitalized?"

"What was the problem that caused the hospitalization, and approximately how long were you hospitalized?" (if relevant, What was the treatment?)

Major Illness

Ask about specific diseases when appropriate. Many heart disease patients forget they also have diabetes.

Many patients have been told in the past that their blood pressure was too high, but they never followed up with a physician.

Trauma

"Have you ever had any major injuries?"

Surgery

"Have you ever had any surgeries?" (Because many surgeries are done on an outpatient basis, you cannot assume the patient has not had surgery if she denies hospitalization. If told of any surgeries when asking about hospitalizations, be sure to say, "aside from what you told me already?" or the SP will think you're not listening.)

PAMH<u>R</u>FOSS: Review of Systems (ROS)

Review of systems is the time to ask screening questions. It is the time to see if there are other major problems that you have not yet uncovered. You can ask about any organ system that you feel is relevant, but focusing on 3 systems is sufficient for most cases. Depending on the relevance, select 3 of the following:

HEENT

"Do you get headaches?"

"Have you had any visual changes?"

"Do you have any trouble with your ears?"

"Do you get nosebleeds?"

"Do you have any throat pain or soreness?"

"Do you have any difficulty swallowing?"

Constitutional (an especially important category to ask because it helps you understand if the problem is systemic, i.e., an infection or cancer)

"Have you been having fevers?"

"Have you been feeling warmer or colder than usual?"

"Do you sweat or have chills at night?"

"Has there been any change in how much you sleep or eat?"

"Are you feeling fatigued or weak?"

Increased sleep may be due to depression, hypothyroidism, sleep apnea, medication, or illegal drugs.

Decreased sleep may be due to anxiety, depression, hyperthyroidism, medication, illegal drugs, or mania.

Respiratory

"Do you get shortness of breath?"

"Do you wheeze?"

"Do you cough up sputum?"

Cardiac

"Do you ever feel your heart beating rapidly (have palpitations)?"

"Do you have any trouble with your heart?"

"Do you have any difficulty exercising, walking up stairs, doing your regular activities?"

Gastrointestinal

"Have you had any change in your bowel habits?"

"Do you have any trouble with diarrhea or constipation?"

"Has your weight changed any?"

"Have your eating habits changed in any way?"

Note: It is common for vegans to develop vitamin B12 deficiency.

Have prepared by Test Day the short differential for weight gain and weight loss:

Weight gain: depression, hypothyroidism, an edematous state (heart failure, chronic liver disease, or chronic renal failure), and eating disorder (not common as a CS exam case)

Weight loss: neoplasm, depression, anxiety, hyperthyroidism, chronic illness, use of an illegal drug, a chronic illness, and eating disorder

Urinary

"Have you had any changes in your urinary habits?"

"How often do you urinate?"

"How many times do you get up at night to urinate?"

"Do you have any burning with urination?" "Any blood?"

"Is the stream weak?"

"Do you ever lose control of your bladder?"

If the chief complaint is dysuria, all of the questions above are asked in the HPI.

Musculoskeletal

"Do you have joint pain anywhere in your body?"

PAMHRF<u>O</u>SS: Family History

The family history is relevant only if the diagnosis you are considering has a genetic or familial component. Do not ask the family history if it isn't relevant. If you do need a family history, make a transitional statement first. "Now I will ask you about your family's health." Then, ask as many of the following questions as appropriate.

"Does anyone in your family have what you have?"

"Does anyone in your family have high blood sugar?" "High blood pressure?"

"Does anyone in the family have any serious illness?"

If a serious illness or death is mentioned in the family history, a simple compassionate statement is always appreciated by the patient: "I am sorry to hear that."

PAMHRF<u>O</u>SS: Obstetrical and Gynecology History

Relevance to the HPI is the key for asking questions about the obstetrical and/or gynecological history. Remain sensitive about a patient's culture and privacy. Iron-deficiency—the most common reason for anemia—is related to the combined effects of menses and pregnancy.

Obstetrical History

How to determine a patient's GPA status:

G = number of times pregnant

Ask, "How many times have you been pregnant?"

P = number of live births; any pregnancy that ended at 20 weeks or later, even if it did not result in a live birth

Ask, "How many times have you given birth?"

A = any pregnancy that ended prior to 20 weeks, including miscarriages, induced abortions and ectopic pregnancies

Ask, "Have you had any miscarriages or elective abortions?"

Gynecological History

Components of a comprehensive gynecological history are the following:
- Regularity of menses
- Cramps/pain with menses
- Flow amount (can be assessed by determining number of sanitary pads/tampons used per day) and number of days the flow is heavy)
- Cycle length
- Age of menarche/age of menopause
- Spotting between cycles
- Vaginal discharge
- Last Pap smear

Suggested questions are:

"When was your last menstrual period?"

"Was it normal?"

"Any change in your period recently?"

"Do you have a period every month?" "How long between periods?"

"Are you regular? How many days do you use pads or tampons? How many pads or tampons per day?" (Note: In the United States, average total number for a menstrual flow is 12/menses.)

"When did you start having periods? When did you stop menstruating? Have you had any bleeding or spotting since menopause?"

"Any mood swings or irritability around your period? Anything else?"

PAMHRFO<u>SS</u>: Sexual History

The sexual history or parts of the sexual history are needed only if relevant to the case, especially if you think the patient could have a sexually transmitted disease, could be pregnant, or if female, has lower abdominal pain. Also, ask yourself if sexual function could be compromised by the diagnoses you are considering. Examples of this are angina precipitated by sexual intercourse or erectile dysfunction caused by depression, diabetes, or beta blockers.

It is important that you not be nervous when asking these questions. Practice them over and over until you can ask them without embarrassment.

Standard sexual history questions are the following:

"Are you sexually active?"

"Are your partners men, women, or both?"

"How many sexual partners have you had in the last 6 months? in the last 10 years?"

"Do you use birth control, and if so, what type? always or sometimes?

(if a female patient takes oral contraceptives, you should still need ask about use of condoms because OCPs do not protect against sexually transmitted diseases)

"Have you ever had a sexually transmitted infection?"

"Have you ever been tested for HIV or AIDS?"

"Do you have any concerns about sexual function?"

Be sure to listen to the patient's answer and consider that most of these questions may not be needed, unless they somehow relate to the chief complaint or your differential diagnosis.

PAMHRFOS<u>S</u>: Social History

The social history is a unique part of the history. It is important because some social behaviors increase the patient's risk for certain diseases. Smoking for many years increases a patient's risk for chronic obstructive lung disease, lung cancer, coronary artery disease, peripheral vascular disease, abdominal aortic aneurysm, and cerebral vascular disease. Long-term alcohol abuse increases a patient's risk for liver disease.

This is also the time to ask about sick contacts (for instance, if the patient has a sore throat, find out if anyone she lives with also has a sore throat).

The social history also helps strengthen the physician/patient bond. The patient will feel that you are really taking an interest in him. You will rarely need to take a complete social history. However, the following components may be important, depending on the chief complaint and your postulated differential diagnosis.

- Tobacco
- Alcohol
- Recreational drugs
- Diet
- Exercise
- Occupation/work life
- Home life

Ask, when appropriate, a question about intimate partner violence: "I ask my patients whether there are problems or conflicts at home?"

Depending on the case, ask about parts or all of the social history.

Tobacco

An efficient way to determine smoking history is to ask the following:

Doctor: "Have you ever used tobacco products?"

Patient: "Yes, I smoked for 30 years and stopped last week. I also stopped using cigars and chewing tobacco last week."

Incorrect: "Do you smoke?"

If you asked the same patient, "Do you smoke?" he may reply "No," because he quit last week. In that case, you would miss the entire tobacco history!

If the patient has a disease that is caused or exacerbated by smoking, it is helpful to know the total lifetime exposure.

Pack-Years = (number of packs per day) x (number of years)

So 20 pack-years could mean 20 years at 1 pack per day or 40 years at one-half pack per day.

If the chief complaint is that the patient wants to receive smoking cessation help, you will need to know when he started to smoke, what he has tried to do in the past to stop, and what methods of quitting have and have not been successful for him.

Alcohol

Ask about alcohol use if it is appropriate for the case. An effective way to ask about alcohol use is the following:

Doctor: "Do you drink alcohol?"

Patient: "Yes."

Doctor: "What do you like to drink and how much do you drink in a typical day?"

Quantify the number of alcoholic beverages your patient drinks in a day—it doesn't matter if it is beer, whisky, vodka or wine. If a man or woman drinks one glass of wine (or anything else) daily with dinner, you do not need to ask any further questions. These patients do not need counseling and they certainly do not need to be asked the CAGE questions.

If, however, you suspect alcohol abuse (a man who consumes more than 2 drinks a day OR a woman who consumes more than 1 drink a day OR anyone who binges on the weekends), then the CAGE questions would be appropriate to determine if the patient is abusing alcohol.

CAGE Questionnaire

Ask the following questions if you suspect the patient has a problem with alcohol:

1. "Have you ever felt you should Cut down on your drinking?"

2. "Have people Annoyed you by criticizing your drinking?"

3. "Have you ever felt bad or Guilty about your drinking?"

4. "Have you had a drink first thing in the morning to steady your nerves or get rid of a hangover? (Eye opener)?"

Two positive responses suggest the patient may have an alcohol abuse problem. Counseling and support services should be offered to the patient.

Courtesy of Dr. John Ewing. "Detecting Alcoholism: The CAGE Questionnaire, JAMA 252: 1905-1907, 1984."

Recreational (Illegal) Drug Use

The correct way to ask about drug use is the following:

Doctor: "Do you or have you ever used recreational drugs?"

Patient: "Yes."

Doctor: "What do you use?"

Patient: "Cocaine, when I can get it."

Doctor: "How do you take it?"

Patient: "I smoke it."

Doctor: "When did you last use?"

Patient: "About 20 minutes ago."

If a patient uses recreational drugs, you should identify the specific substances, routes used (ingested, smoked, snorted, or IV), and date of last use. A patient may be willing to quit; ask if an attempt has been made and what method has been tried.

SPs do make an effort to avoid using slang words in their speech. If you don't understand the street name of a recreational drug, it is fine to ask the patient.

Patient: "I use coke sometimes."

Doctor: "Is that cocaine?"

Patient: "That's right, Doc."

Common Names for Recreational Drugs

Alcohol: booze, brews, brewskis

Amphetamines: speed, crank, crystal meth

Cannabis: hash, hashish, dope, pot, reefer, bud, ganja, weed, grass

Cocaine: blow, coke, toot, nose candy, crack

Downers: generic street name for benzodiazepines or barbiturates

Heroin: horse, brown sugar, smack

Phencyclidine: PCP, angel dust

'Roids: anabolic steroids in general

Exercise

Asking about exercise is appropriate when a patient comes in for a general checkup or a periodic physical exam, but not when the visit is for an acute problem.

Occupation/Work Life

A patient's occupation and occupational exposures may be clues to the cause of symptoms. A high stress level at work can be the foundation for symptoms. A coal miner who is short of breath may have pneumoconiosis.

Marital Status/Home Life

Asking about home life provides noteworthy social information, particularly if you suspect intimate partner violence:

Doctor: "Do you live alone or with others?" (If "with others" but the patient doesn't clarify, ask what their relationship is.)

Patient: "My wife and our 3 teenagers."

Doctor: "Is there any stress at home?"

Patient: "No, just the usual stuff with kids."

THE PEDIATRIC HISTORY

Infants and children do not participate in the CS exam. A parent, grandparent, or guardian will present the child's history in person or through a telephone conversation. Review all components of the chief complaint and HPI, as noted in previous sections, with the parent or guardian. Ask about pregnancy and delivery, and then about the child's growth and development, nutrition, immunizations, and progress in school. (The first thing on the diagnostic workup should be the physical exam.)

THE PATIENT WITH A PSYCHIATRIC DIAGNOSIS

Two psychiatric illnesses common in the United States are depression and anxiety reaction—with or without panic attacks. Both are diagnosed by a physician's clinical judgment. Psychiatrists order a panel of laboratory studies to ensure the symptoms are not related to the presence of a chronic illness (see below). When you consider either of these diseases, use the following hints and mnemonics as a guide. (Note: A patient with schizophrenia may also be seen on the exam.)

Depression

For an accurate diagnosis of depression, one of the symptoms must be **depressed mood or loss of interest in carrying out pleasurable activities**. Symptoms are worse in the morning and should be present more days than not for at least 2 weeks. Two excellent screening questions are the following:

"Do you feel sad a lot lately?"

"Have you lost interest in most of your activities lately?"

Patients with depression often present with a somatic symptom as the chief complaint, e.g., headache, insomnia, abdominal pain, musculoskeletal pain, or not feeling right. Appetite and weight may increase or decrease. Insomnia or hypersomnia may be present. Common precipitants of depression are financial problems, work issues, change in a relationship, a medical problem, loneliness, or, moving.

If depression is suspected, ask the following questions:

S = "How has your Sleep been lately?"

I = "How is your level of Interest?"

G = "Do you have any feelings of Guilt?"

E = "How has your Energy level been lately?"

C = "How is your Concentration?"

A = "How is your Appetite?"

P = "Do you feel restless or slowed down?" (Psychomotor)

S = Have you thought about killing yourself or ending your life? (People may not understand the word *suicide*.) (There is an increased risk of Suicide when there is (1) a definite plan, (2) previous attempt that failed, and (3) family history of suicide in a first-degree relative.)

Anxiety Reaction

Anxiety is "too much worry or nervousness." While everybody worries a bit, it becomes a problem when it interferes with daily functions. Patients often present with somatic symptoms: fatigue, muscle tension, chest discomfort, trouble catching breath, or palpitations. They have difficulty concentrating at work or school and trouble sleeping soundly. Patients appear nervous, jittery, and worried.

"Are you worrying or more nervous than usual?"

"What are you worrying about?"

"Is your worry keeping you up at night, making it difficult to concentrate, or eat?"

A **panic attack** is severe worry accompanied by the physical symptoms of palpitations, sweating, shaking, trouble breathing, chest discomfort, and lightheadedness. As noted above, anxiety overlaps with depression; if you suspect one, always ask about the other and list both in the differential diagnosis.

Focused Physical Exam

5

The physical exam is sharply focused on the patient's chief complaint, the symptoms identified during the HPI, and your generated hypotheses. To perform a targeted physical exam, you must have a well-considered differential diagnosis and knowledge of which physical findings would be expected for each condition included in the differential. Because of the time constraint imposed by the Step 2 CS, it is critical that you keep your exam focused.

GENERAL POINTS

- Standardized patients (SPs) are diligently trained to simulate the illness being portrayed.
  - Physical findings can be imitated and enhanced by the application of stage makeup.
  - Actors with actual abnormalities, as well, can be placed into the setting of the case. A person with a known cardiac murmur can reliably simulate a patient with infective endocarditis.
    - Therefore, consider all detected abnormalities as real.
- You are **not permitted** to do the following exams: female breast, pelvic, rectal, genital (including evaluation for inguinal hernia), or corneal reflex.
  - Instead, list a necessary exam for any of these regions in your diagnostic plan.
  - If synthetic models are used for these exams, instructions will be provided.
- At the appropriate time, tell the patient you are going to conduct the exam, wash your hands or use hand sanitizer, and proceed.
  - Drape the patient with care; never examine through clothing.
  - Make sure the patient removes socks if you are going to examine the feet.
  - As you examine a region, describe what you are doing, e.g., "I am examining your ears to see if you have an infection."
- For women, ask the patient to assist you when examining the anterior thorax, heart, and lungs.
  - She can lift her breast to enable you to look for and palpate the apical impulse. Instruct her to move her bra.
- If the patient is fearful of an exam due to pain, say, "I know you are in pain, but it's important that I examine you. I'll be gentle and quick and I'll let you know exactly what I'm going to do before I do it."
  - Assist the patient into the best position to help relieve some of the pain (i.e., adjust the table up or down).
- It's perfectly appropriate to ask questions about the history during the physical exam.
- Allow 3 to 4 minutes to perform the physical exam. Your main objective is to thoroughly examine the target area and use the remaining time to examine other areas related to your differential.

EXAMPLE PHYSICAL EXAM

A 73-year-old man presents with left-sided chest pain, nausea, diaphoresis, and palpitations.

Differential diagnosis:

- Acute coronary syndrome
- Pulmonary embolus
- Pneumothorax
- Pneumonia
- Costochondritis

Physical exam checklist:

- ❏ Washed hands prior to exam
- ❏ Palpated left chest wall for reproducible tenderness
- ❏ Looked and palpated for apical impulse
- ❏ Palpated apical impulse
- ❏ Auscultated heart in all 4 cardiac areas
- ❏ Examined lungs (6 areas in back, 4 areas in front)
    - A. Inspection for symmetrical expansion
    - B. Tactile vocal fremitus
    - C. Percussion
    - D. Auscultation
- ❏ Inspected for JVD
- ❏ Evaluated peripheral pulses
- ❏ Inspected calves for swelling, tenderness

In this case, the cardiac and lung exams were relatively thorough because cardiac and pulmonary diseases were high on the differential diagnosis list. A neurologic exam was not necessary (especially if, during the history-taking section, the patient denied having any numbness/tingling or weakness).

- In your Patient Note, comment on the general appearance. If the patient above was visibly uncomfortable due to the left-sided chest pain, you could write, "Patient uncomfortable secondary to pain."
- Accept the vitals as being correct. Do not repeat them unless you are instructed to do so by the Doorway Information.
- Try to start with the most relevant organ system first, and do it completely. Then, examine other organ systems that are relevant to the differential diagnosis.

FOCUSED EXAMS BY SYSTEM

HEENT (Head, Eyes, Mouth, Ears, Nose, and Throat) Exam and Neck/Thyroid Exam

Do HEENT and Neck exams when there are complaints of:

- Headache
- Head trauma
- Ocular problems (visual disturbance, eye pain)
- Ear problems (tinnitus, vertigo, hearing loss)
- Nasal problems (rhinorrhea, epistaxis, sinus pain)
- Pharyngitis, voice changes, jaw pain
- Fatigue

Only perform the relevant components of the HEENT and Neck/Thyroid exams depending on your differential diagnosis. To conduct the exam, do the following:

 Head

- Inspect for trauma, scars, hair changes, other relevant abnormalities
- Palpate for tenderness — *HA complaint*

 Eyes

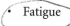 *Vision*
— acuity
— visual fields

- Inspect sclera/conjunctiva for color; pupils for size, shape, and symmetry
- Inspect visual acuity with the Snellen chart
    - Ask patient to cover left eye and read the smallest possible line on the chart; check acuity in both eyes
- Peripheral vision (visual fields):
    - Have patient cover the eye that is not being tested; it is crucial that patient look straight ahead and not at your fingers
    - Rapid method: bisect the pupil horizontally and vertically, creating 4 small quadrants
        ° First, wiggle your fingers in both upper (superior) quadrants, then in both lower (inferior) quadrants, asking patient to point to which fingers are moving
    - Now repeat the same maneuver with other eye, checking all 4 visual fields
- Central vision, macular degeneration:
    - Check with finger in front of nose
- Check extraocular movements
    - Ask patient to look straight ahead and follow your index finger; make a wide "H" in the air, and ask patient to follow with the eyes
    - This will check all of the extraocular movements and check for nystagmus
- Pupillary light reflex: check direct response (constriction of the illuminated pupil), as well as consensual response (constriction of the opposite pupil)
- Check accommodation: it is easier to view the pupil dilate rather than constrict because most irises are dark brown
    - Place your finger 12 inches from eye, then ask patient to look into the distance; the pupil will dilate

dilate looking to the distance

- Inspect the fundus:
    - Dim lights in room
    - Remove ophthalmoscope from holder and make sure unit is turned on
    - Shine light on your hand, adjusting light color and diameter (set lenses at zero)
    - Ask patient to stare at a point on the wall
        ◦ Coming in from the side and holding instrument in right hand, use your right eye to examine patient's right eye
        ◦ Then hold instrument in left hand and use your left eye to examine patient's left eye

Ears

- Assess hearing:
    - With eyes open, rub together thumb and index finger by each ear to determine if the patient can hear sound.
    - Then, with eyes closed, start rubbing fingers at a distance, moving toward the ear.
    - Ask the patient to tell you when the sound is audible (normal is 6 inches from the pinna).
- Inspect the external ear for abnormalities. Palpate the ear, tragus, pinna, and mastoid area for tenderness.
- Inspect the canal and drums.
    - Remove the otoscope from its holder and turn light on.
    - Put on a new speculum; secure it tightly
    - Gently move pinna superiorly (up) and posteriorly (back); this maneuver straightens the cartilaginous section of the canal
    - Gently, by direct visualization, place tip of speculum into the external auditory meatus
    - Gently introduce the speculum while looking through the lens; once the tip is in the ear canal, do not move the otoscope in any plane as that would cause discomfort to the patient
- Do Rinne and Weber tests only if there is hearing loss on history or physical exam.
    - **Rinne:** Place vibrating tuning fork on mastoid process. When patient no longer hears it, move to external ear and determine if patient can still hear the vibration.
    - **Weber:** Place vibrating tuning fork on center of forehead. Check if sound is equal in both ears.

Use of a Tuning Fork to Determine the Cause of Hearing Loss: Sensorineural Versus Conductive

Diagnosis	Hearing	Rinne	Weber
Normal	Normal	AC > BC	Equal
Conductive loss	Decreased	BC > AC	Louder on the side with the hearing loss
Sensorineural loss	Decreased	AC > BC	Louder on the normal side; softer on the side with the hearing loss

Nose

- Inspect the external nose
- Palpate nose and sinuses (frontal and maxillary)
- Inspect nasal turbinates with a light source

Oral cavity and throat

- Inspect with a light source
- Inspect the tonsillar fossae and oropharynx; gently use a tongue depressor, keeping it anteriorly to prevent a gag reflex
- Examine oral cavity, tongue, and oropharynx

Neck Exam

- Untie the gown, moving it inferiorly to below the clavicles. Explain to the patient the necessity for improving exposure.
- Inspect the neck for any visible abnormalities.
- If there are musculoskeletal symptoms, examine the muscles of the neck for tenderness and perform a range of motion.
- Examine the neck for lymphadenopathy:
  - Using both hands simultaneously, palpate with the finger pads of the 3 middle fingers while moving in a circular motion. Begin in the posterior neck inferior to the occiput (occipital nodes), moving to the mastoid processes (postauricular nodes), anterior to pinnae (preauricular nodes), inferior to mandible (submandibular nodes), and inferior to chin (submental nodes).
  - Move fingers along the sternocleidomastoid muscle (superficial cervical nodes), along the anterior edge of the trapezius (posterior cervical nodes), and in the angle formed by the sternocleidomastoid and clavicle (spraclavicular nodes)

Thyroid Exam

- Ask patient to swallow (offer water if needed); observe thyroid gland movement.
- Go around the back (or stay in front, whichever you prefer), and using the finger pads of your 3 middle fingers, palpate the thyroid gland below the cricoid cartilage on both sides
- Ask patient to swallow again, feeling the thyroid gland slip under your fingers.
- Hold the left side of the thyroid gland stationary while you palpate the right. Check for nodules, tenderness, or enlargement. Then do the same on the other side.
- Check for associated abnormalities like skin, hair, reflexes and heart rhythm changes. Also examine for myxedema and tremor.

Suggested Phrasing for HEENT Exam

Action	Suggested Phrasing	Comments
Palpation of head	"I need to press lightly on your head."	
Palpation of sinuses	"Now let me press lightly on your face."	
Palpation of ears	"Now I'll press around your ears. I need to pull up on your ears now."	
Palpation of lymph nodes	"I need to check your neck for swollen glands."	"Lymph nodes" is medical terminology.
Otoscope Eyes Nose Oral cavity and throat	"Please pick a point on the wall and look at it. I'm going to check your eyes." "I'm going to check your nose." "Say 'ah.'" (Note: Letting the tongue rest on the floor of the mouth rather than protruding it actually improves visibility.)	
Weber	"Now I need to check your hearing. I'm going to put this tuning fork on your head. Tell me if it sounds the same in both ears."	
Rinne	"I'm going to put the tuning fork behind your ear. Can you hear this? Tell me when you can't hear it any longer." Once the patient can no longer hear it, move tuning fork anterior to ear and ask, "Can you hear it now?"	
Thyroid Auscultation of gland Palpation of gland	"Now I need to check your neck area." "I'm going to press lightly on your neck, so I'll need you to swallow. Would you like some water? Okay, let me get it. Please take a drink and hold it until I ask you to swallow."	The word "thyroid" may be considered medical terminology. Demonstrates empathy to offer water to help patient swallow more easily. If patient doesn't want water, don't insist.
Palpation of skin	"I need to check your skin."	Check for myxedema.
Hair brittleness	"I need to check your hair."	
Check for tremors	"Please hold out your hands like this and close your eyes."	Demonstrate how patient should hold hands.

Neurologic Exam

A complete neurologic exam is not possible during the CS 2 exam because of its length; different parts are appropriate, depending on the differential diagnosis.

- If a patient presents with symptoms consistent with cerebral vascular disease or subdural hematoma, focus the exam on detecting an upper motor neuron lesion.
  - This could include cranial nerves, motor and light touch of all 4 extremities.

[Handwritten notes in top margin: DM2 — vibration, light 7-touch, sharp, position, DTRs]

- If a patient with diabetes mellitus presents with symptoms of peripheral neuropathy, focus the exam on testing the 4 sensory modalities—light touch, pain (using toothpicks on the CS), vibration, and position—and the deep tendon reflexes on both upper and lower limbs.
  - Listen for a carotid bruit in the presence of symptoms of a transient ischemic episode (attack), i.e., TIA.
  - Carpal tunnel syndrome is the most common entrapment neuropathy. Know the sensory distribution of the median nerve and the small muscles of the hand innervated by the nerve.
    - Tapping the flexor retinaculum with a finger or reflex hammer will elicit dysesthesias in the sensory distribution of the median nerve (Tinel's sign).

Components of the Neurologic Exam

Not all components will be necessary.

Mental status
- Orientation (level of consciousness, orientation to person, place, and time) *AO×3*
- Concentration (serial sevens or spell "world" backwards)
- Memory (remember 3 things); ask to repeat after a few minutes

Cranial nerves
- CN I: not tested
- CN II: vision (acuity, visual fields, PERRLA)
- CN III, IV, VI: extraocular movements
- CN V: sensation on face (all 3 areas) and motor component (clench your teeth)
- CN VII: close eyes tightly; smile; raise eyebrows
- CN VIII: hearing testing
- CN IX, X: look for symmetry of uvula
- CN XI: trapezius and sternocleidomastoid movement and power
- CN XII: protrude tongue

Upper limbs (compare one side to the other)
- Test tone and strength by passively flexing and extending
- Test biceps muscles and wrist extensors against resistance

Lower limbs (compare one side to the other)
- Test tone and strength by passively flexing and extending at the joints.
- Test flexors of the hip (iliopsoas) and dorsiflexors of the feet (tibialis anterior) against resistance.

(Continued)

Components of the Neurologic Exam (*Cont'd*)

Reflexes (not all are needed for every patient)
- Biceps
- Triceps
- Brachioradialis
- Patellar
- Achilles
- Babinski

Biceps (C5, C6)

Patient's arm should be partially flexed at the elbow with palm down. Place your thumb or finger firmly on the biceps tendon. Strike with the reflex hammer so that the blow is aimed directly through your digit toward the biceps tendon.

Triceps (C6, C7)

Flex patient's arm at the elbow and pull it slightly across the chest. Strike the triceps tendon above the elbow.

Brachioradialis-Supinator Reflex (C5, C6)

Patient's hand should rest on the abdomen or the lap, with the forearm partly pronated. Strike the radius 1-2 inches above the wrist. Watch for flexion and supination.

Quadriceps-Knee Reflex (L2, L3, L4)

Briskly tap the patellar tendon below the patella. Note contraction of the quadriceps with extension at the knee. A hand on the patient's anterior thigh lets you feel this reflex. The quadriceps are the strongest muscle in the body so expect a forceful response.

Gastrocnemius-Ankle Reflex (primarily S1)

- If patient is sitting, dorsiflex the foot at the ankle. Strike the Achilles tendon. Watch and feel for plantar flexion.

- If patient is lying down, flex one leg at both hip and knee and rotate it externally so that the lower leg rests across the opposite shin. Then, dorsiflex the foot at the ankle and strike the Achilles tendon.

Plantar response (L5, S1) and the Babinski response

With an object such as a key or the wooden end of an applicator stick, stroke the lateral aspect of the sole from the heel to the ball of the foot, curving medially across the ball. Use the lightest stimulus that will provoke a response. Note movements of the toes, normally flexion. Dorsiflexion of the big toe, often accompanied by fanning of the other toes, constitutes a Babinski response.

Eliciting the Reflexes

Sensory

- Demonstrate sharp/dull
- Tell patient to close eyes
- Test sensory regions related to presenting complaint
- Repeat with light touch
- Test position sense using the big toe
- For vibration sense, begin with the first metatarsal joint of each foot, moving to bony prominences proximally until the patient perceives vibration

Cerebellar

- Finger to nose
- Heel to shin
- Rapid alternating hand movements
- Gait: ask patient to walk across room

Specific tests

Romberg sign (to assess the posterior columns, i.e., position sense, in a patient with unsteady gait/balance): Ask patient to stand with feet together. (Be ready to assist in case patient begins to fall.) First, test stability with patient's eyes open. If patient is steady with eyes open, repeat with eyes closed.

Kernig sign (when meningitis is suspected): With patient lying supine flex a knee, extend the leg on the thigh. A positive test is flexion of the neck as you extend the leg.

Brudzinski sign (when meningitis is suspected): If positive, gently flexing the neck results in flexion of both knees.

Babinski sign: Gently stroke lateral border of plantar surface of foot beginning at the heel and moving across the metatarsalphalangeal joints (see diagram). A positive test is dorsiflexion of the big toe with the other toes separating and dorsiflexing (extending, moving upward).

Suggested Phrasing for Neurologic Exam

Action	Suggested Phrasing	Comments
PERRLA	"I need to check your eyes."	
Funduscopic	"Now I need to shine the light so I can examine the back of your eyes. Thank you."	If patient resists, say, "I need to look at the blood vessels back there to make sure they're not damaged. It's extremely important for your safety."
Cranials **3, 4, 6**	"Please follow my finger without moving your head."	
5	"I'm going to touch your face lightly. Do you feel this? Now please close your eyes. Do you feel this? How about this? Is it the same?"	Do for all 3 branches. Then say, "Now you may open your eyes."
7	"Please close your eyes tightly and resist my trying to open them."	If any sentence is difficult for you to pronounce, just demonstrate the action and say, "Do this."
7 **9, 10** **11** **12**	"Please smile and show me your teeth." "Please open your mouth so I can see your throat." "Now shrug your shoulders." "Now please stick out your tongue and move it from side to side."	

Upper limbs
Muscle testing
	"First I will check the tension in your muscles by moving them."
	"Now I will test your strength."
	  (Remember "MRS": Muscles).
	"Extend your arms with palms up."
	  Close your eyes.
	"Make a muscle and resist me from pushing your arms down."
	"Extend your wrists and resist me from pushing them down."
	"I will tap on your arms for reflexes." (Reflexes)
		Remember "MRS":
		Muscles

Reflexes
Sensory
  Light touch
	"Now I need to tap on your arms."
	"Now I need to check your sense of touch."
	"Now I'm going to touch your hands lightly. Tell me if you feel it. Does it feel the same? Okay, now close your eyes."
		Reflexes
		Sensation
		  Repeat for 3 points on hand then say, "Okay, you may open your eyes now."
		  Repeat for 3 points on hand. Then say, "Please open your eyes."

Sharp and dull	"Now I need to check your sharp and dull sensation. This is sharp. This is dull. Please close your eyes and tell me what you feel. Which is this? And this? How about this?"	
Vibration	"I'm placing this tuning fork on your 4th finger. Please close your eyes. Do you feel the vibration? Please open your eyes."	
Position sense	"Now I'll be moving your 4th finger. Please close your eyes, this is up, this down; now tell me if it is up or down? You may open your eyes."	

(Continued)

Suggested Phrasing for Neurologic Exam (*continued*)

Action	Suggested Phrasing	Comments
Lower extremities	"I need to check your leg strength. May I raise the sheet? Thank you."	
Muscle testing	"First I will check the tension in your muscles by moving them."	Test patellar and achilles.
	"Now I will test your strength."	
	"Extend your entire lower limb, resisting as I try to push down."	
	"Now move your foot toward your nose, resisting as I try to push down."	
	"I will tap on your arms for reflexes."	
Reflexes	"Now I'm going to tap on your legs."	Tap in 2 areas.
Babinski	"Now I need to tickle (or scratch) your feet lightly."	
Sensory		
Light touch	"I'm going to touch your legs lightly. Tell me if you feel this. Please close your eyes.	Repeat for 4 points. "Please open your eyes."
	Do you feel this? This? Does it feel the same?"	
Sharp and dull	"Now I need to check your responses to sharp and dull touch. This is sharp. This is dull. Please close your eyes. Which is this? How about this?"	Repeat for 4 points on feet. "Please open your eyes."
Cerebellar		
Finger to nose	"Please touch your nose with this finger, then touch mine."	Hold up your own index finger to demonstrate.
Heel to shin	"Please do this. Do the same with your other leg."	
Gait	"Now I need to see how you walk. Let me pull out the footstool. May I help you step down? Please walk to the other side of the room and back. I'll stay with you."	Physically assisting the patient shows empathy.
Romberg	"Please stand with your feet together, hold out your arms and close your eyes." (*demonstrate this*) "I will be standing beside you to prevent you from falling."	Demonstrate action. Such phrases show empathy.
Kernig	"I need to uncover your leg. I'm going to bend your knee and then straighten it. Tell me if it hurts."	
Brudzinski	"I'm going to gently flex your neck and will stop if there is pain. Just relax while I do this."	

Pulmonary Exam

Do a pulmonary exam when there are complaints of cough, shortness of breath, wheezing, chest pain, and symptoms of upper respiratory infection. Do a thorough exam of the lungs whenever there are symptoms of pulmonary disease. Since you will be behind the patient at times and he won't be able to see what you are doing, it is important to let the patient know in advance before you do each step.

Inspection

- Presence of dyspnea or use of accessory muscles

Palpation

- Examine for chest wall tenderness
- Assess symmetrical expansion by placing hands on thorax during a deep inspiration
- Check tactile fremitus (say "99"); compare side-to-side; examine 6 regions posteriorly:
  - Adjacent to medial aspect of each scapula
  - At each lung base
  - In both mid-axillary lines at midpoint of the thorax

Percussion

It is critical to compare the right side to the left.

- Explain to the patient that you are going to untie the gown in back.
- Lay your nondominant hand over the left lung apex; apply pressure and, using your dominant middle finger, tap on the middle finger of the nondominant hand (using a wrist hammering motion with your dominant wrist).
- Percuss the left lung apex, then immediately compare this percussion note (which is a hollow sound) to the percussion note of the right lung apex.
- Next, move to the mid-portion of the left lung and compare the note to that of the right.
- Finally, come down to the left lung base and compare the note to the right lung base. This way, both lungs have been done symmetrically.

Auscultation

Auscultation of the lungs is strongly recommended when there are primary pulmonary symptoms. Always compare side to side. Let the patient inhale/exhale before moving to the next area.

- Listen to the 6 posterior regions. Ask the patient to open her mouth and take deep, slow breaths in and out. Make sure you listen to a full inspiration and expiration in each region.
- Start with the left apex and compare it to the right.
- Move to the mid-portion of the left lung and compare it to that of the right.
- Finally, compare the left base to the right. Note any difference you hear on the left side compared to the right. (The patient may "fake" taking a deep breath when you listen to the right lung; if that happens, write "No breath sounds in right lung" in your Patient Note. This could happen with a pneumothorax case.)
- Examine 4 regions of the lungs anteriorly. Perform fremitus, percussion, and auscultation comparing both sides.
- Now compare the left thorax lateral to the heart—lingual segments—with the right anterior thorax—middle lobe; perform fremitus, percussion and auscultation.

Suggested Phrasing for Pulmonary Exam

Action	Suggested Phrasing	Comments
Posterior chest	"May I untie your gown? I need to check your lungs."	
Respiratory excursion	"Please take a deep breath. Cross your arms in front and sit up straight."	
Tactile fremitus	"Please say 99. Again."	Repeat at each level.
Percussion	"Now I'm going to tap on your chest."	
Auscultation of lungs	"I need to listen to your lungs. Please breathe normally in and out through your mouth. Okay, thank you."	If you can't hear the breath sounds adequately, ask the patient to breathe deeply in and out.
Anterior chest	"I need to lower your gown."	
Tactile fremitus	"Please say 99. Again."	Repeat at each level.
Percussion	"Now I'm going to tap on your chest."	
Auscultation of lungs	"Let me listen to your lungs. Please breathe in and out through your mouth. Thank you."	
Auscultation of heart	"Now I'll listen to your heart. Please breathe normally."	

Cardiovascular Exam

Do a cardiovascular exam when there are complaints of chest pain, palpitations, shortness of breath, loss of consciousness, or pedal edema.

- Examine external jugular vein. Place the table at a 30° angle. Ask the patient to turn his head slightly to the left. Shine a light source obliquely over the area of the external jugular vein on the right side of the patient's neck.
- Ask female patients to assist by raising the left side of the gown to below the bra/left breast. Then have them lift the bra slightly while you say, "I am looking for your heart beat and will touch the area to identify where the beat is located."
- Auscultate the heart beginning at the apical impulse (mitral valve). Move your stethoscope horizontally to the left parasternal line (tricuspid valve). Lower the gown to where it was located.
- Ask the patient to lower the upper edge of the gown to the level of the bra/breasts. Listen over the second left intercostal space to the pulmonic valve and then to the aortic valve over the second right intercostal space.
- Examine peripheral pulses
  - If appropriate, listen for a carotid bruit at the bifurcation of both common carotid arteries (located anterior to sternocleidomastoid on a horizontal line drawn from the thyroid notch). Do not palpate the bifurcation site because one may activate a baroreceptor within the carotid sinus, which is located superior to the bifurcation in the wall of the internal carotid artery and cause bradycardia or a vasovagal response.

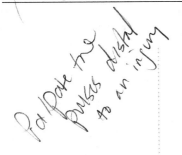

Palpate the pulses distal to an injury

– When appropriate, examine the peripheral pulses in the lower limbs: start with posterior tibial, and dorsalis pedis. If these are not palpable then move proximally to the popliteal then femoral arteries.

– Palpate pulses distal to an acute injury. For example, if an 18-year-old boy fell off his scooter and hurt his left elbow, palpate the radial and ulnar arteries.

Suggested Phrasing for Cardiovascular Exam

Action	Suggested Phrasing	Comments
Sitting up		
Carotid bruit	"I need to listen to your neck sounds. Breathe in and out 3 times, then hold your breath."	
Palpation of pulses	"I'm going to check your pulses."	
Edema	"I'm going to check your legs for swelling."	
Inspection and palpation of apical impulse	"Please raise your gown. I need to examine your heart beat."	For women, you may need to ask, "Please lift your breast. Thank you."
Auscultation of heart	"I need to listen to your heart."	Leave gown untied.
Auscultation of lungs	"While you're sitting up, let me listen to your lungs."	Three levels posterior
Lying down		
JVD	"Please look to the left. I need to take a look at your neck."	Adjust table for JVD and pull out extension.
Costochondral tenderness	"Now I need to press on your chest. Any pain?"	Maintain eye contact.
Epigastric tenderness	"Now I need to press on your stomach area."	

JVD = jugular venous distention

Abdominal Exam

Do an abdominal exam when there are complaints of the following:

- Abdominal pain
- Diarrhea
- Constipation
- Nausea
- Vomiting
- Weight loss or decreased appetite
- Hematochezia
- Jaundice
- UTI symptoms

- Hematuria
- Pelvic pain
- Pregnancy
- Abnormal vaginal bleeding
- Sexual dysfunction
- Hematemesis

Inspection:

- Properly drape the patient by lifting the gown to just above the costal margins; move the sheet to above the inguinal ligaments. Inspect for distension, scars, rashes, bruises or any other abnormality; tell the patient that you are inspecting the skin.
- Auscultate for bowel sounds prior to palpation and percussion. Listen 3 seconds in each quadrant.
- Gently palpate the abdomen in all 4 quadrants. Do not use excessive force, as this may harm the SP.
- If indicated, evaluate for the presence of an enlarged spleen or liver by asking patient to take a deep inspiration when palpating inferior to the costal margins. The normal spleen is not palpable; a normal liver may descend 1-2 cms with deep inspiration. Once again, do not use excessive force!

  worried about hepato or spleno megaly

- Note any areas with rebound tenderness. Watch the patient's face for an indication of discomfort or pain.
- The percussed span of the liver in the right midclavicular line correlates with the true size of the liver. Normal span is 8-12 centimeters; taller women and men have longer spans. Percuss the superior border by moving inferiorly from the resonance of normal lung to dullness. Then percuss the inferior border by moving superiorly from abdominal tympany to dullness. During the CS 2 exam, it is impossible to accurately measure the span of the liver because of the presence of the bra. For women, percuss the inferior border only.
- To evaluate for the presence of ascites percuss, start at the umbilicus moving to the flanks.

  Only if worried about liver failure

- If you are considering partial rupture of an abdominal aortic aneurysm, listen for a bruit over the surface projection of the abdominal aorta—xyphoid process to superior and to the left of umbilicus.

Other tests

- **Murphy's sign**: palpate inferior to the right costal margin
  - Cessation of respiration during deep inspiration is a positive Murphy's sign.
- **Rovsing's sign**: palpation of the left lower quadrant increases the pain in the right lower quadrant

  Rovsing's sign

  - CVA tenderness is present during an episode of acute pyelonephritis.
  - Lightly tap the costovertebral angle; tenderness is often severe
- List a pelvic or rectal examination on your diagnostic plan.

Suggested Phrasing for Abdominal Exam

Action	Suggested Phrasing	Comments
Inspection	"Let me take a look at your stomach area.	The word "abdomen" is considered medical terminology. Use "stomach area," "belly," or "tummy." If you notice any scars or abnormalities, ask about them.
Auscultation	"Now I need to listen to your belly."	Warm up your stethoscope head before touching patient with it.
Light palpation	"I need to press lightly on your stomach area."	Examine painful areas last.
Percussion	"I need to tap on your tummy."	
Rebound tenderness	"Now I need to press in on your stomach area. Tell me if it hurts more when I press in or let go."	
CVA tenderness	"I'm going to gently touch your back. Let me know if it hurts."	
Special test for cholecystitis Murphy's sign	"I need to press in on your stomach area. Please take a deep breath and let me know if it hurts."	

Musculoskeletal Exam

Musculoskeletal pain is a common reason Americans visit physicians. Symptoms are usually located in one region or one joint. Lumbosacral strain and intervertebral disc protrusion or herniation—in either cervical or lumbar regions—are common. Straight-leg raising test will exacerbate pain if there is sensory root compression. Examine the sacroiliac joints and gait when evaluating a patient with low back pain.

Do a musculoskeletal exam when there are complaints of:

- Joint pain
- Extremity pain
- An acute injury
- Decreased range of motion
- Weakness
- Fatigue
- Any rheumatology case

SI joints
pain
from
straight leg raise

To assess the presence of the most common disc herniations or protrusions, use the following guidelines.

DISC /ROOT	REFLEX	MUSCLE/SENSATION
C6-C7 C7	Triceps	Wrist drop/extensors; second & third fingers
L4-L5 L5	Patellar	Foot drop/tibialis anterior; great toe
L5-S1 S1	Achilles	Gastrocnemius; lateral foot

- Always compare the affected side to the normal one
- Palpate the joint distal and proximal to the complaint joint
- Inspect the joint or region for erythema or swelling; palpate for warmth and tenderness. Performing an active range of motion with the patient facilitates the exam.

Because it is often challenging to identify the exact location of an abnormality, shoulder and neck are examined as one region, regardless of where the pain is located. After testing the active range of motion of shoulder joints, test internal and external rotation passively.

- Elbow region are examined for the presence of epicondylitis, when appropriate
- Wrist/hand is evaluated for carpal tunnel syndrome
  - Tinel: tap the wrist at the flexor retinaculum (over the median nerve)
  - Phalen: patient places dorsum of hands together facing downward
- Hip joints are examined passively to more accurately test range of motion (internal rotation, external rotation, flexion, and extension if concerned that the patient has arthritis of the hip (patient must lie on abdomen, face down, or stand/extend the leg backward)
- Knee joints: anterior and posterior drawer, medial and lateral collateral ligaments, McMurry's [rewrite as full sentence; see samples above]
- Ankle joints and feet are examined as one region, actively and passively.
  - Palpate the plantar fascia to assess for the presence of plantar fasciitis; note the increase in tenderness at the point the fascia inserts on the calcaneus
  - If appropriate, perform a limited neurologic examination of the affected region
  - Assess vascular status (pulses) in the affected region. Musculoskeletal and neurologic exams have areas of similarity.

Suggested Phrasing for Musculoskeletal Exam

Action	Suggested Phrasing	Comments
Always let the patient know beforehand when you're going to untie, raise, or lower the gown. Tie the gown when your examination is complete.		
Wrist pain Inspection	"Let me take a look at your wrist and other joints."	Paraphrasing what the patient has told you shows care and concern.
Palpation	"I know you have pain on this side, so let me start with the normal side first. Now let me check this side."	
Active range of movement	"Now I need to see how your joints are moving. Let me start with the one that doesn't hurt."	
Passive range of movement	"I will now gently move your joints."	
Muscle testing for UE	"Do this. Don't let me push in. Don't let me push out. Do this. Don't let me push up. Don't let me push down. Do this. Don't let me squeeze your fingers together. Do this. Squeeze my fingers as hard as you can. Thank you."	Don't say "ouch!" if the patient squeezes too hard.
Reflexes for UE	"Now I need to tap on your arm."	Tap in 3 areas on each hand.
Sensory	"Now I'll check your sensation."	
Light touch	"I need to touch your hands lightly. Tell me if you feel this. Please close your eyes. Do you feel this? How about this? Does it feel the same?"	Repeat for 3 points on hand. "Please open your eyes now."
Sharp and dull	"Now I'll check your sharp and dull touch. This is sharp. This is dull. Okay, please close your eyes. Which is this? Which is this?"	Repeat for 3 points on hand. "You may open your eyes now."
Carpal tunnel evaluation		
Tinel	"I need to tap on your wrists. Let me start with the one that doesn't hurt."	
Phalen	"Do this. Let me know if it hurts."	Demonstrate action.
Shoulder pain Inspection	"Let me take a look at your shoulder and other joints."	
Palpation	"I know you said it hurts, so I'll start with the other one. I need to untie your gown. Okay, now I'm going to press on your neck. Any pain? Now your shoulder blade [or] Now here. Any pain? Now let me do the same on the other side. Let me tie your gown back."	
Range of movement	"I need to check on your shoulder movement. With the hand that doesn't hurt, do this. This. This. Now with the other hand, go only as far as you can. Do this. Do this. This. Thank you."	Repeat for other shoulder.
Muscle testing for UE	"I need to check your arm strength. Do this. Don't let me push in. Don't let me push out. Do this. Don't let me push up. Do this. Don't let me push down. Don't let me squeeze your fingers together. Do this. Squeeze my fingers as hard as you can."	
Reflexes for UE	"Now I need to tap on your arms."	Repeat for 3 areas.
Sensory for UE Light touch	"I need to check your sensation. May I pull up your sleeves? Thank you. Now I'm going to touch your hands lightly. Do you feel this? Please close your eyes. Do you feel this? And this? Does it feel the same? Do you feel this? This? Does it feel the same?"	Besides the 3 points on hand, check deltoid area. Repeat for 4 points. "Please open your eyes."
Sharp and dull	"Now let's check sharp and dull. This is sharp. This is dull. Which is this? This?"	Repeat for 4 points. "Please open your eyes."

UE = upper extremity; LE = lower extremity

(Continued)

Suggested Phrasing for Musculoskeletal Exam (*continued*)

Action	Suggested Phrasing	Comments
Lower back pain		
Inspection	"Let me take a look at your other joints."	
Palpation	"I need to press on your back. Now I'm going to press over here. May I untie your gown?"	
Muscle testing for LE	"I need to check your leg strength. Push out. Pull back. Push on the gas [or] Push down. Pull up."	
Reflexes	"Now I'll tap on your legs."	
Sensory for LE		
Light touch	"I need to check your sensation. I'm going to touch your legs lightly. Do you feel this? Now please close your eyes. Do you feel this? This? Does it feel the same?"	Repeat for 4 points. "Open your eyes."
Sharp and dull	"Now I need to check your sharp and dull touch. This is sharp. This is dull. Okay, please close your eyes. Which is this? This?"	Repeat for 4 points. "Open your eyes."
Babinski	"Now I need to tickle your feet [or] I need to scratch your feet."	
Gait	"I need to see how you walk. Let me pull out the footstool. May I help you down? Please walk to the other side of the room and back. I'll be nearby."	
Range of motion	"Please bend down and try to touch your toes. Now twist from side to side [or] Do this. Now, lean back."	Demonstrate twisting.
Knee pain		
Inspection	"Let me check your knees."	
Palpation	"I know you said this knee hurts, so I'll start with the other one. Let me lift the sheet so I can press on your knee."	
Range of motion	"Let's see how your leg moves."	
Muscle testing for LE	"Let's check your leg strength. Push out. Pull back. Push on the gas [or] Push down. Pull up."	
Reflexes	"Now I need to tap on your legs."	
Sensory for LE		
Light tough	"I need to check your sensation. I'm going to touch your feet lightly. Do you feel this? Please close your eyes. Can you feel this? How about this? Is it the same? Do you feel this? This? Is it the same?"	Repeat for 4 points. "You can open your eyes now."
Sharp and dull	"Now let's check your sense of sharp and dull. This is sharp. This is dull. Okay, please close your eyes. Which is this? This?"	Repeat for 4 points. "Please open your eyes."
Pulses	"I need to check your pulses."	
Knee joint effusion	"Let's see if you have any swelling. Okay, now the other knee."	
Anterior/posterior drawer sign	"I need to push and pull on your knee. Okay, now the other one."	
McMurray	"I'm going to push down on your knee and move your foot. Okay, now the other knee."	
Collateral strain	"I need to push on your knee. Now the other one."	

Patient Note

6

Immediately after each patient encounter in Step 2 CS, you will be asked to type (on a computer) a Patient Note similar to the medical record you would compose after seeing a patient in a clinic, office, or emergency department.

The Patient Note is an important component of the ICE score and the only component of the CS exam graded by a physician. You will be graded using a global rating scale and not a specific checklist. Your note must therefore reflect an intelligent logical approach to patient care and differential diagnosis.

PATIENT NOTE LOGISTICS

We encourage you to become familiar with the Orientation and Practice Materials for Step 2 CS, including Patient Note interactive simulations and *samples of Patient Notes* that are available at usmle.org. Your Patient Note practice should be conducted in format available on that web page, which is the same format that will be used on the day of your exam.

You will be required to type all your Patient Notes. Stay within the space allotted for each section. There are characters as well as line limits for each field on the Patient Note screen as follows:

- **History:** 950 characters, 15 lines
- **Physical Examination**: 950 characters, 15 lines
- **Diagnosis**: 100 characters for each diagnosis
- **History Findings and Physical Examination Findings**: 100 characters per field
- **Diagnostic Studies**: 100 characters per study recommendation

You may add rows to History Supporting Findings, Physical Examination Supporting Findings, and Diagnostic Studies sections up to a maximum of 8 rows each. The Patient Note screen that appears during the actual exam will have a status bar for both history and physical examination, indicating how many characters have been used.

A blank sheet of paper is provided for writing brief notes during the actual USMLE encounters. These notes are not read and therefore not factored into your overall Patient Note performances.

PATIENT NOTE ORGANIZATION

To the best of you're ability attempt to use correct grammar and sentence structure. An occasional misspelled word—as long as it does not change the meaning of that word—could be acceptable. Practice spelling words that are commonly misspelled—*pneumonia, abscess, inflammation,* and *ischemia*—and any other common medical terms that give you difficulty.

Step 2 Clinical Skills

A good Patient Note, in particular good history and physical, will involve typing what you **asked of** the patient, what **exam** you did, and what you have **observed during encounters**. Remember, if no physical exam is performed (as in a phone case), leave the physical exam section blank.

There are 4 components to every Patient Note:

- History
- Physical Examination
- Differential Diagnosis (1–3 rows)
- Diagnostic Workup (1–8 rows)

CLINICAL SKILLS EVALUATION
PATIENT NOTE

HISTORY: Describe the history you just obtained from this patient. Include only information (pertinent positives and negatives) relevant to this patient's problem(s).

PHYSICAL EXAMINATION: Describe any positive and negative findings relevant to this patient's problem(s). Be careful to include *only* those parts of examination you performed in *this* encounter.

DATA INTERPRETATION: *Based on what you have learned from the history and physical examination*, list up to 3 diagnoses that might explain this patient's complaint(s). List your diagnoses from most to least likely. For some cases, fewer than 3 diagnoses will be appropriate. Then, enter the positive or negative findings from the history and the physical examination (if present) that support each diagnosis. Lastly, list initial *diagnostic* studies (if any) you would order for each listed diagnosis (e.g. restricted physical exam maneuvers, laboratory tests, imaging, ECG, etc.).

DIAGNOSIS #1:

HISTORY FINDING(S)	PHYSICAL EXAM FINDING(S)

(+) Click to add row(s)

DIAGNOSIS #2:

HISTORY FINDING(S)	PHYSICAL EXAM FINDING(S)

(+) Click to add row(s)

DIAGNOSIS #3:

HISTORY FINDING(S)	PHYSICAL EXAM FINDING(S)

(+) Click to add row(s)

DIAGNOSTIC STUDIES

(+) Click to add row(s)

Copyright ©2012 by the National Board of Medical Examiners (NBME®) and the Educational Commission for Foreign Medical Graduates (ECFMG®).

History

The history section contains all of the information subjectively given to you by patients. This includes the "story" about their chief complaint (HPI), all of the **pertinent positives/negatives** from the ROS, PMH, meds, allergies and **pertinent social/family history**.

- Focus sharply on HPI and include pertinent positives and negatives
- Consider and document only relevant components of PMH
- To get a point for the CC, 3 components are needed: age, gender, complaint (i.g. 68 yo M c/o chest pain)
- Common abbreviations can be used to save time and space in your Patient Note. Refer to **Appendix** to see an extensive list of potential abbreviations.

History of Present Illness (HPI) and Past Medical History (PMH):

The history section should include all information that you have been collecting during the encounters using the mnemonics. **PMH** includes all pertinent information with regards to the individual patient, their chief complaint and your differential diagnosis. It includes serious illnesses/significant hospitalizations/surgeries, medications, allergies, and pertinent social/family history. See chapter 3 for details on history taking.

When typing the history component of your Patient Note, to save time and characters, consider using phrases rather than sentences:

- *64 y/o woman c/o substernal chest pain*
- *8/10 in intensity, heavy, crushing, constant pain*
- *Started 1 hour ago while watching TV*
- *Radiates to L arm and jaw*
- *Nothing makes it better. Worse with exertion*
- *(+) SOB, diaphoresis*
- *(−) syncope, fever, cough, palpitations, leg swelling*
- *No previous episodes*
- *No Rx or OTC meds, NKDA*
- *Denies hx of htn, dm, or high cholesterol*
- *(+) smoker (30 pack years), denies ETOH and drugs*
- *No family hx of heart disease*

For Past Medical History and Social History (PMHx/PSHx), "*not relevant*" is acceptable and requires no further detail.

Physical Examination

For the physical examination, start by listing the vitals (given on doorway information) and the general appearance. Record the focused physical examination that you performed, including both positive and negative findings.

- First, familiarize yourself with the normal exams of each tested systems.
- Then, think about how you would document an abnormality that may be present.

When typing your Patient Note, do not type components of the history and physical that you did not conduct. In cases where the patient is not present—phone case or surrogate—leave the physical exam section blank. Read carefully your doorway information; you will be given clear instructions on parts that you are not expected to do.

Physicians grading your notes are more concerned with your ability to communicate your objective physical findings than with your format or punctuation. Write phrases rather than sentences.

When considering how to take notes, follow this sample for general headings:

GA: general appearance

VS: vital signs

Chest or **Lungs:** chest

ABD or **Abd:** abdomen

HEENT: head, eyes, ears, nose, throat

Neuro: neurologic exam

CV: cardiovascular

UE & LE: upper extremity and lower extremity

Vital Signs

Vital signs (given on doorway information) should be noted on every Patient Note. If a patient's chief complaint is cough, and you noted on the doorway information that there was fever, **make sure to record or interpret** the fever (i.e., febrile) on your Note. That would be a pertinent vital sign most likely supporting your differential diagnosis.

If all vital signs are normal, you could use the abbreviation **WNL** (within normal limits). If only one vital sign is abnormal, you could state **VS: WNL except BP 150/100.**

In the presence of fever, respirations 30/min, pulse 120/min, and blood pressure 90/60 mm Hg, these would all be pertinent vital signs and should be recorded in the beginning of your physical examination component. For example:

- VS–90/60, p 120, RR 30, afebrile
- Vitals–120/80, p 86
- Vital signs–normal or VS WNL
- VS–T 40, BP 120/70, p 84
- Vitals normal except BP 180/90

Height and weight should be noted if relevant to the case; that would include a general physical or periodic health exam, pre-employment physical, life insurance, or any other time you think it may be relevant. For example:

- Wt–100 kg
- Weight 155 lbs; height 5 ft 2 inches

General Appearance (GA)

This is the place to describe the patient you saw sitting in front of you as you began your physical exam. Comment on any unusual behavior observed. It's fine if you have some components of psychiatric or mental status here in particular if your differential diagnoses are psychiatric. Some examples:

- GA: NAD (no acute distress)
- GA: in [mild/moderate/severe] distress from [pain/SOB]
- GA: no distress, A&O x3 (alert and oriented times 3)
- GA: pt is pacing the room in [pain/anger/rage]
- GA: dirty, torn clothes; smells of beer (or other body odor)
- GA: quiet, flat affect; will not make eye contact
- GA: track marks on arms, multiple bruises

Skin

Skin could be treated as a system on its own. Describe the anatomic location of any encountered color changes, tenderness, warmth, as well as the pattern of any flat/raised lesions as precisely as possible. Some examples:

- Skin: multiple blue/red macules on upper and lower ext in sun-exposed areas. Warm & tender. No streaks.
- Skin: jaundice (or Skin: yellow powder on face)
- Skin: [track/needle] marks on both arms

HEENT

While typing the note for each organ system you can follow the same outline that you are already familiar with from the physical examination section.(Inspection, Palpation, etc.). There is no need to type subheadings for eyes, ears, etc. The abbreviation HEENT stands for:

Head

Eye

Ear

Nose

Throat

A normal **HEENT** is given below:

HEENT: normocephalic/atraumatic (NC/AT), nontender. PERRLA. Fundi–red reflex intact, EOMI. Fundoscopy Nl. No papilledema. Vison WNL. No visual defect. TMs, pharynx–WNL. Nasal turbinates not congested, no nasal discharge. No tonsilar enlargements, erythema, exudates, vesicular lesions. Neck supple. Lymph nodes NL, (or no LAD), thyroid not enlarged.

If abnormalities on the **HEENT** are found, be as specific as possible in describing them. For example:

- HEENT: tender, pre-auricular node and pinna, (-)redness,(-) swelling
- Head: deformity, tender with epistaxis from right nostril
- Head: b/l tenderness [maxillary sinus, cheek]
- Head: fine, thin hair. No exophthalmos [diaphoretic, sweating], no thyroid enlargement. [Tenderness, deformity, crepitus] to [nose, cheek, maxilla, jaw, zygoma, orbit, forehead]

Further examples of **HEENT** note-writing:

- PERRL: (pupils equal, round, reactive to light)
- PERRLA: (the "A" stands for "and accommodation")

- PERRLA: sclera clear, EOMI (extraocular movement intact). Extraocular muscles intact except [R 6th nerve palsy, R lateral gaze deficit].
- Visual fields intact, or R [temporal, nasal] visual field deficit
- Visual acuity: VA–20/20 OU (OU = both eyes, OS = left eye, OD = right eye). VA: 20/200 R eye, counting fingers 5 ft L eye.
- Visual acuity: L eye light perception only, OD–20/200. Fundi: flat (no papilledema), or Fundi: Not visualized, or Fundi–NL red reflex.

For nose, be as specific as possible:

No nasal discharge and/or good air entry b/l, or b/l thick yellow discharge or nasal septum [intact/perforated]

For ears:

- *Pinna NL. TM WNL b/l (tympanic membrane normal bilaterally)*
- *R TM red bulging, L NL. (Right tympanic membrane is red and bulging, L tympanic membrane is normal)*
- *TMs both with [perforation/holes] b/l*

For throat:

- *Pharynx [clear, red, with exudates, NL]*

Teeth

- *[Dentition/Teeth], [poor/normal]*

Thyroid

- *Thyroid: [nontender/tender], [normal size/enlarged]. No nodules.*
- *Nontender, NL size, no nodules, trachea in midline; or Tender, enlarged, trachea shifted L*

Lymph nodes

You may examine a patient for cervical, axillary, and femoral triangle (inguinal) lymph nodes.

- *Lymph nodes: not swollen or tender - or no LAD*
- *Hard, tender supraclavicular lymph node*
- *Diffuse lymphadenopathy (seen with mononucleosis)*

You may also list the particular nodes that are swollen and tender, such as the following: [submandibular, submental, preauricular, postauricular, anterior cervical, posterior cervical, supraclavicular, subclavicular] adenopathy.

Chest/lungs

Remember to do a complete chest exam (inspection, palpation, respiratory excursion, tactile fremitus, percussion, and auscultation) and document all your findings. Again, document *everything* you do so you can maximize your score.

Normal chest exam:

- *Chest appears NL, nontender, NL resp, excursion, fremitus, percussion NL and equal b/l. Lungs clear to auscultation bilaterally; CTA b/l.*
- *Chest without deformity, skin WNL. Lungs clear to A&P b/l (A&P means "auscultation and percussion").*

Abnormal chest exam:

- *Inspection: Increase AP diameter, or pursed-lip breathing, or chest with deformity or [ecchymoses/bruise] R flank, or thoracotomy scar*
- *Palpation: Tenderness on [R lat 8th rib, L CVA, lumbar spine, R costochondral margin]. Be as specific as possible about the area of tenderness.*
- *Respiratory excursion: Poor respiratory excursion or paradoxical chest wall excursion*
- *Fremitus: [increased/decreased] fremitus [R/L] [base/midlung field/apex]*
- *Percussion: [dull/hyperresonant] percussion [R/L] [base/midfield/apex]*
- *Auscultation: [decreased/absent] breath sounds [L/R]. Or you may have heard abnormal sounds: [wheeze, rhonchi, rub, rales] [L/R] [base/midlung/apex]*

Cardiovascular

Normal cardiovascular exam:

- *Regular rate & rhythm (RRR); apical impulse not displaced(PMI); S1, S2-WNL; no rub/gallop/murmur (MRG); no JVD, clubbing, or edema. No carotid artery bruits. Peripheral arterial pulses palpable in lower limbs.*

For the normal person, you could write **"No JVD"** or **"JVP NL"**; either notation is correct.

In fact, you could also write **"CV : S1, S2 WNL, RRR, no RMG."**

If abnormalities are found on the cardiovascular exam, be as specific as possible. Most SPs will have expectedly a normal CV exam.

For pulse:

[R/L] [radial/brachial/femoral/popliteal/DP/PT] pulse [absent/decreased/NL/bounding]

For point of maximal impulse (PMI):

PMI displaced

If you felt the apex, you can describe its location, e.g., PMI at anterior axillary line, 8th rib.

For heart rate and rhythm, the grading scale for murmur is as follows:

- 1/6 = faintest murmur
- 2/6 = soft murmur
- 3/6 = loud murmur
- 4/6 = very loud murmur with palpable thrill when you check PMI
- 5/6 = heard with stethoscope partly off the chest
- 6/6 = heard with stethoscope off the chest

Note

An irregularly irregular heart rhythm is often atrial fibrillation.

[**RRR, irregular irregularly rhythm**] + **gallop rhythm** (Write this when you hear an S3 or S4 heart sound.)

[**1/6, 2/6, 3/6, 4/6**] [**diastolic/systolic**] **murmur** is the basic notation for murmur. A murmur can be pansystolic, early, or late.

Abdomen

Document the parts of physical examination that you have conducted: inspection, auscultation, percussion, and palpation.

Normal abdomen exam:

ABD: symmetric nl appearance, BS present, no bruits heard, liver span in right MCL = 10cm; spleen not palpable; no abd. mass. No tenderness.

Document all additional tests performed even if they are normal:

Murphy's sign: absent; no CVA tenderness; no flank dullness; negative Psoas and Obturator, Rovsing's and rebound

Accurately describe abnormalities:

- *Skin: record scars or other changes indicating correct anatomical delimitation*
- *Palpation: note location of direct or rebound tenderness by region or quadrant; indicate anatomical location of tests performed in the abdomen if they are positive*

Bowel sounds will always be present. Record with accuracy what **is present**, not what **should be present**.

Neurological

Think about the entire neurological exam and write down the parts that you have performed. If abnormalities are found, be as specific as possible in describing them.

Complete normal neurologic exam:

Neuro: A&Ox3. CN 2 - 12 NL. Sensation to light touch, position sense and vibration sense intact all 4 ext. on lower ext NL B/L. Motor 5/5, DTR 2/4, B/L all 4 ext. Gait–WNL. No Kernig or Brudzinski. Neck supple. Straight leg raise negative B/L. Romberg negative. Coordination intact. No dysmetria or dysdiadochokinesia. Babinski–nl B/L.

For mental status abnormalities, if the patient knows only her name but not the place or date:

A & O x 1 (or Alert and oriented to person only)

For cranial nerves, you can interpret the physical finding or just describe it:

Pt points tongue out to L = L 12th nerve palsy

Entire R side of face is weak, pt cannot close R eye = R peripheral 7th CN lesion

For sensation, describe where the patient is experiencing numbness. Sensations described/ tested are sharp, dull, vibration and position sense.

- *[Decreased/No] light touch below knee B/L; no position sense L toe, R lower ext. WNL*
- *Numbness R ulnar nerve distribution (Numb 5th digit R hand.)*

Motor

Motor function is traditionally graded on a 5-point scale.

0/5	flaccid
1/5	just a flicker of movement
2/5	so weak that the patient cannot overcome gravity
3/5	can overcome gravity
4/5	somewhat weak
5/5	normal

- *Motor: 3/5 RUE, other ext NL describes someone with a weak R arm and the other 3 extremities normal.*

You may also use regular language to describe the degree of weakness. For instance:
- *Motor: [Mild/Moderate/Severe] weakness RUE*
- *Motor: Pt with [dense paralysis/0/5] entire R side of body, L side WNL*

Reflexes

Reflexes are traditionally graded on a 4-point scale.

0/4	no reflex
1/4	decreased
2/4	normal
3/4	somewhat hyperreflexic
4/4	clonus (very hyperreflexic)

- *DTR: 1/4 brachial B/L (decreased reflex brachial DTR both sides)*
- *DTR: R brachial & patella 4/4, L 2/4 (patient who is hyperreflexic on R side of the body)*

Gait
- *Gait: ataxic if unsteady or patient unable to walk*
- *Romberg: positive if patient cannot perform test and falls to one side*

Meningeal Signs
- *Meningeal signs: + stiff neck, + Kernig, + Brudzinski*

Straight Leg Raising
- *Straight leg raise: + R, neg on L is how to chart the straight leg raise test*

Extremities

Depending on the case, you may need to comment on joints in general (lupus or rheumatoid arthritis) or on specific joints (an acute injury). Some examples:

- R wrist-swollen, erythematous, decreased active or passive ROM
- Joints-no swelling/ erythema / tenderness/ full ROM
- L elbow-no swelling/ red/ tender/ limited ROM
- MCP's and PIP's-red, swollen and tender bilaterally
- If a patient presents with right knee problems, for example, while considering a differential diagnosis for knee pain, take into consideration as well hip problems that can refer to the knee and present as knee pain.
- A sample Patient Note for normal lumbosacral and lower extremities is presented below:
- Lower back: no obvious deformities or signs of trauma; no spinous process or paraspinal tenderness and full ROM to flexion, extension and lateral rotation.
- Lower extremities: ROM WNL, motor 5/5 , B/L, DTR 2+ (patellar, Achilles) sensation intact to sharp and dull B/L
- Gait: WNL
- Peripheral Pulses: 2+ DP, PT
- Normal Psychiatric Mental Status Exam

Below is the documentation of the normal version of the psychiatric examination:

- **GA:** Patient appears well-groomed, alert and oriented to person, place, and time (A&O x 3), Speech fluid and goal-directed; Recent and remote memory intact; Attention and concentration unimpaired; Mood euthymic; affect c/w mood; No abnormal perceptions: hallucinations, delusions, or paranoia; No suicidal/homicidal ideation or intent; Judgment/insight are intact.

DIFFERENTIAL DIAGNOSIS

An important component of the Patient Note is the differential diagnosis filled in with all supporting data. There are 3 available spaces for differential diagnosis.

- List diagnoses in order from **most likely** to **least likely**, typing only one diagnosis per line.
- Your diagnoses should be written **based on the hypotheses generated from the introductory information**, and then further refined during the history-taking and physical examination.
- Your diagnoses must be supported by entering the positives and negative findings from the history and physical examination.
  - Include the relevant supporting factors in the appropriate spaces of your Patient Note (up to 8 rows for each diagnosis).
  - Attempt to document 8 total findings for the first diagnosis, and 4 for each additional diagnosis chosen. Since time is limited, you are not expected to fill in 8 rows of history findings and 8 rows of physical findings for every differential diagnosis.

Helpful Tips for Differential Diagnosis

- Write the most likely diagnosis first.
- Use only those abbreviations listed on the usmle.org website. If you are unsure about the abbreviation, type out the full name.
- Write diseases, not symptoms
  - Congestive heart failure, not shortness of breath
- Include only diagnoses that can be supported by the patient's symptoms, past medical history and/or physical exam findings.
- You may list fewer than 3 diagnoses in certain cases. Make sure that every diagnosis listed can be supported with history and physical findings.
- "Noncompliance with medicine" and "medication side effect" can be legitimate diagnoses.

DIAGNOSTIC WORKUP

The last component of the Patient Note includes immediate plans for a diagnostic workup. Here, you will carefully correlate the list of all immediate diagnostic tests that you will perform to further confirm your differential diagnosis. Guidelines for writing the workup include the following:

- You are given up to 8 rows on this section; if more then 8 tests are appropriate for a given case, group similar tests as 1 row such as: blood & urine tests, radiologic tests.
- Include prohibited physical exam maneuvers that are relevant to the case.
- Do not mention treatments, counseling, hospitalizations, referrals, or consultations
- Use acceptable abbreviations
- For a case with no workup, write "*No studies indicated*"; do not leave it blank.
- Do not list test panels or groups, e.g., LFTS but instead list AST, ALT
- You will not receive credit for listing allowed physical exam maneuvers you would have done if the encounter had been longer

PATIENT NOTE TIME MANAGEMENT

If you leave the patient encounter early, you may use the additional time for typing the note. On rare occasions the computer may malfunction. If that happens, you will be asked to hand-write the Patient Note by using the same format. Go to usmle.org and familiarize yourself with the Patient Note format and **practice, practice, practice!** Here are a few tips to help improve your practice performance:

- Use either the mouse or tab to move to the next box
- To highlight a single word, drag or double click the left mouse button. To highlight an entire line drag using the left mouse button (select all will select the whole section, not just the wanted line).
- To copy/paste, highlight and then use the right mouse button or CTRL C and CTRL V
- Leave out commas when it does not interfere with understanding
- When justifying the differential diagnosis, enter relevant information under the first differential and then copy and paste what is relevant into the other diagnosis.

Remember that **time is of the essence**; listing **phrase format** (examples given through this chapter) is preferred over narrative paragraph to save time. To earn more points, we suggest that you type the following first:

- Chief complaint and HPI
- Relevant PMH
- Differential diagnosis with justification
- Diagnostic studies
- Physical examination

Depending on the time you have left, add additional information collected during the encounter from the PMH.

PRACTICE CASE

Now that you have completed the chapter on the Patient Note, you should be able to write an excellent note. First, go back to the **original practice case in chapter 2**, and review the history and physical examination. Then go to **usmle.org** and type your Note for the case. Remember to set a timer for the 10 minutes allotted.

Once you have completed your Note, compare it to the one below. Given the time constraints of the exam, your Note will be somewhat shorter.

PATIENT NOTE FOR PRACTICE CASE: SEVERE ABDOMINAL PAIN

Patient Note

History

CC: 35 yo F c/o severe abdominal pain

HPI: RLQ, x6hrs, 10/10, sharp, stabbing, sudden, constant, progressive, no radiation, no precipitating factors. Aggrav by movement and deep breaths. No relief with advil. + vaginal spotting and nausea. No vomiting, diarrhea, anorexia, fever, vag discharge or urinary changes.

PMH: no h/o CC or trauma. h/o UTI, PID. Hosp/surg for appendectomy

ObGyn: G0P0, LMP 6 wks ago

Meds: advil prn, No Rx. NKDA.

FHx: No h/o CC or illnesses

SH: Sexual active with bf, 20 M partners x 10 years, occ condoms, HIV not tested. No tobacco or rec drugs. Occ EtOH

Physical Examination

VS: 98.6 F, RR: 19/min, HR 100/min, BP 120/78 mm Hg

General: Pt lying in fetal position in acute distress

Abd: RLQ scar. +BSx4Q, tympanic x4Q, soft, not distended. + RLQ tenderness, + rebound. No CVA tenderness. No hepato-splenomegaly

Data Interpretation

DIAGNOSIS 1. ECTOPIC PREGNANCY

History Support	Physical Exam Support
Acute RLQ pain	Afebrile
LMP 6 wks ago	RLQ tenderness
Vag spotting	Rebound
Nausea	No CVA tenderness
h/o PID	
Age 35	
h/o ruptured appendix	
No vag D/C	

Diagnosis 2. Ovarian Torsion/Ruptured Ovarian Cyst

History Support	Physical Exam Support
Acute RLQ pain	Afebrile
h/o ruptured appendix	RLQ tenderness
Progressive sharp pain	Rebound
Nausea	No CVA tenderness
LMP 6 wks ago	
Vaginal spotting	
No vag D/C	

Diagnosis 3. PID

History Support	Physical Exam Support
h/o PID	RLQ tenderness
Multiple sex partners	No CVA tenderness
Inconsistent condom use	
Abdominal pain	
Vag spotting	
Nausea	

Diagnostic Studies

Pelvic/rectal exam
B-HCG, CBC w diff, ESR, CRP
Pelvic U/S with color flow Doppler
Cervical swab: GC, chlamydia, C/S

Differential Diagnosis

7

Each standardized patient (SP) encounter requires test takers to exhibit capable data-gathering through the history and focused physical examination. The task is to generate hypotheses, leading to the establishment of a differential diagnosis.

Generating hypotheses begins outside the exam room with the posted patient information: patient's age, chief complaint or reason for the visit, location of the encounter, and vital signs, e.g., *a 58-year-old man presents to the clinic with chest pain of several hours' duration.*

This "doorway information" sets the stage for the encounter by enabling you to think of possible common diagnoses before the start of the encounter. Possible common reasons for chest pain in a 58-year-old include:

- Acute coronary syndrome, MI
- Acute coronary syndrome, unstable angina
- Pneumonia
- GERD
- Costochondritis

If this patient presented with fever, the initial list of hypotheses might be:

- Pneumonia
- Pleuritis
- MI
- Costochondritis

Once inside the exam room, pursue a line of questioning mindful of the diagnoses you are considering. Continue generating hypotheses while you add or remove possible diagnoses. Return to the chief complaint and chronology. Careful consideration of hypotheses will lead to a productive and sharply focused physical exam.

During the examination, continue asking questions about the history of present illness (HPI) as you identify abnormalities. The list of hypotheses will have changed from the time you read the doorway information to the point of presenting your ideas with diagnostic and therapeutic plans.

Suppose a 20-year-old man complains of sudden onset shortness of breath and his vitals prior to your entering the room reveal respiratory rate 40/min and pulse 118/min. In that situation, you may generate a differential diagnosis such as:

- Pneumothorax
- Acute allergic reaction
- Asthma attack
- Pulmonary embolus
- Pneumonia

If this patient denies a fever and cough, pneumonia is very unlikely; it will remain at the bottom of your list. If he has a peanut allergy and just ate Thai food for lunch, he may be having an acute allergic reaction. As you complete your history, you'll want to ask about allergies, history of asthma, trauma, and family history.

If this patient is a healthy young man who arrived home yesterday from a European backpacking trip with his friends, pulmonary embolus would be at the top of your differential diagnosis list. The history he would give you might be that he woke up this morning, got out of bed, and suddenly became short of breath. He might also say that he slept the entire flight home because he was so exhausted from hiking every day.

As you can see from the case of this 20-year-old with dyspnea, **pertinent positives** will help support the likely diagnosis for your case. **Pertinent negatives** will either help eliminate a differential totally or make it much less likely to be the primary diagnosis for the case. Asking the right questions and finding the right positives and negatives will help in diagnosis selection and will be used in the patient note as the findings to justify the differentials chosen.

Another example will help solidify this concept:

> A 30-year-old woman complains of fatigue. She admits to recent weight gain and sleeping more hours than she normally did during the past several years. She denies problems adjusting to temperature changes, and any changes in her skin and hair texture.

These facts make it more likely that the diagnosis for the case is major depressive disorder and less likely that it is a case of hypothyroidism. Nevertheless, hypothyroidism should still be used as a differential for this case.

You are also told that she eats a healthy diet that includes red meat and denies heavy menses. Since there is no evidence of anemia, it should not be considered at all for this case.

Finally, stop and review one last time the approach to differential diagnosis. Now return to your patient note for the chapter 2 practice case and be sure that you can identify and understand the relevant positives from history and physical examination. Next, be sure you understand the included examples of pertinent negatives. Recognize that although the patient has a history of PID and current risk factors, it is listed as the third differential since the patient does not have a vaginal discharge or fever. The case facts you use to determine your diagnoses will be the justifications used in your patient note. The more organized your thought process and approach, the easier it will be to write an excellent patient note. Also remember that the selected differentials are not the only possible ones to use for this case. Others to consider would be threatened/incomplete abortion, urinary tract infection, or even endometriosis.

COMMON ERRORS IN THE DIFFERENTIAL DIAGNOSIS PROCESS

Determining the proper differential diagnosis is one of the keys to passing the Step 2 CS exam. Four common errors may occur.

Error 1. Skipping steps in data-gathering

When generating hypotheses, the history is the most important source of information. Fixating on narrow or incomplete data from initial answers can lead to an erroneous line of questioning with failure to elicit more relevant symptoms.

Solution

- Keep the focus on the generated hypotheses.
- Ask questions leading to or eliminating diagnoses. If you ask, "What other symptoms have you had?," the SP will respond with, "What do you want to know, doctor?"
- Ask about other concerns.
- Always ask for clarification of the events in the HPI.
- Listen carefully to a patient's complete answer before moving on.

Error 2. Using wrong information

Even when you have asked the right question and believe you have eliminated possible diagnoses for the right reasons, it is still possible to use wrong information in your conclusions. For example, in response to the question, "Do you smoke?" the patient says, "No." But had you asked, "Do you use tobacco?" the patient's answer might have been, "I don't smoke, but I do chew."

Solution

- Clarify answers to ensure your correct understanding. ("You said that you have never smoked. Have you used any other tobacco product, like snuff or chew?")
- Consider an answer's completeness and accuracy in the context of the patient's age, gender, or other history. ("You said that both your parents, your siblings, and your wife all smoke, but that you don't. Have you ever used any other tobacco product, like snuff or chew?")

Error 3. Restricting or limiting the problem

It is incorrect to limit or restrict a differential diagnosis based upon preconceived assumptions.

You may prematurely bring closure to a sequence of valid questions. For example, a patient whom you believe is using illegal drugs because of general appearance may lead you away from asking key questions and failing to believe there is no history of illegal drug use.

Solution

- Perform the evaluation based on presented information without making wrong assumptions.
- Be objective in your assessment of the patient's clinical status. Don't let physical appearances influence your establishment of rapport.

Error 4. Giving up on a problem too soon

One of the challenges on the Step CS exam is to have a patient who speaks very little, is angry, or has difficulty communicating information. What behaviors are useful in these situations to enable you to obtain all necessary information?

Solution

- Facilitate communication by encouraging the patient. Repeat or paraphrase what is said to enhance your understanding of the problem. Summaries are extremely helpful, even short ones.

- Use more closed-ended questions; yes/no answers provide information when patients are unable to provide longer answers.
- Most important, demonstrate even more caring and concern about the patient's health with verbal and nonverbal reassurances.
- Start the physical examination earlier than usual. Clues will be present as you examine the patient and continue to ask questions as you move from one region to the next.

Another challenge is generating differentials diagnoses for psychiatric complaints. Two common examples are depression and anxiety.

A differential diagnosis for depression:

- Depression
- Anxiety (depression and anxiety are closely related – if you consider one, list the other)
- Hypothyroidism
- Somatization disorder

A diagnostic plan for depression includes screening tests for common chronic diseases: anemia, renal failure, diabetes mellitus, hypothyroidism, chronic liver disease, or a chronic infection. It is of key importance, and a patient's confidence will increase, if you carefully consider the patient's presenting somatic symptoms. One simple test to assess them; for instance, an abdominal U/S to evaluate abdominal pain can be of therapeutic benefit.

A differential diagnosis for anxiety:

- Anxiety
- Depression
- Hyperthyroidism
- Somatization disorder

A diagnostic plan for anxiety is similar to the one for depression, i.e., screening tests for common chronic diseases: anemia, renal failure, diabetes mellitus, hyperthyroidism, chronic liver disease, or a chronic infection.

Generating an accurate differential diagnosis is a key component of the Step 2 CS exam and an important skill in being a safe and competent physician.

GATHERING DATA TO SUPPORT THE DIAGNOSIS

The following section provides a few common cases, along with the relevant history, physical findings, and appropriate tests that would support a particular diagnosis.

This is intended only as a guide to help you learn how to support your diagnosis and select an appropriate and relevant work up. It is not an exhaustive list.

Case	Diagnosis	HPI	PMH	PE Findings	Work Up
30 yo woman c/o sudden onset severe abdominal pain	Ectopic pregnancy	Sudden onset LLQ, RLQ Severe/progressive Unilateral/ amenorrhea Vaginal bleeding/ Nausea/vomiting Breast fullness Weakness	Previous ectopic pregnancy Fallopian tube pathology and surgery Abdominal surgery In-utero DES exposure PID/infertility Uterine anomalies Smoker Progesterone/ contraception/ IUD	Tenderness Guarding	Pelvic exam Serum quantitative B-Hcg Transvaginal U/S
30 yo woman c/o sudden onset severe abdominal pain	PID	Lower abd pain Gradual or sudden onset Dull and achy/ bilateral Progressive/ Fever Purulent vaginal discharge Nausea/vomiting Anorexia/malaise Onset following menses	Multiple sexual partners Unprotected intercourse Bacterial vaginosis Recent gynecologic procedure HIV	Tenderness Guarding	Pelvic exam NAAT/cultures for chlamydia and gonorrhea Vaginal secretions KOH Transvaginal U/S
30 yo woman c/o sudden onset severe abdominal pain	Appendicitis	Onset Periumbilical/ sharp Progressive to RLQ Anorexia/fever Nausea/vomiting Diarhea/malaise Indigestion/ flatulance	IBD	+ psoas/obturator sign + Rovsing's sign + McBurney's point tenderness	CBC w differential Abdominal U/S CT scan if negative or inconclusive

(Continued)

Case	Diagnosis	HPI	PMH	PE Findings	Work Up
30 yo woman c/o sudden onset severe abdominal pain	Ovarian Torsion	Sharp Intermittent worsening Exercise precipitated Unilateral Radiates to flank, back, and/or groin Fever Nausea/vomiting	Previously resolved episodes Pelvic surgery Ovulation induction		Pelvic exam Pelvic U/S Doppler *assess flow*
30 yo woman c/o sudden onset abdominal pain	Ovarian cyst rupture	Unilateral at onset Diffuse Exercise precipitated Vaginal bleeding Nausea/vomiting Shoulder pain	LMP 2 wks ago (midcycle)	Cullen sign	Pelvic exam Pelvic U/S
45 yo woman c/o right sided abdominal pain *Fat Female Fertile 40*	Cholecystitis	+ Relationship to fatty foods + Radiation to R scapula + Association with N/V + Feverish	OCP use Obese DM Family h/o gallbladder disease + Multiparity	Overweight Fever Tenderness in RUQ Murphy's sign	CBC w/diff Abd U/S AST, ALT, ALP, bilirubin ERCP
Middle age woman with joint pain, swelling of her hands, low grade fever and fatigue for several mos	Rheumatoid arthritis	Symmetric Morning stiffness >1 h Duration 6 w Symptoms improve w/ motion	FH	+ rheumatoid nodules	Anti-cyclic citrullinated peptide ANA, RF Hand/wrist x-ray
Middle age woman with joint pain, swelling of the hands, low grade fever, and fatigue for several mos	SLE	Morning stiffness <1 h Photosensitivity Oral ulcers Alopecia Weight loss *rash* *pleurisy*	FH	Malar/discoid rash	ANA Anti-dsDNA AB Anti-Sm AB Complement level Antiphospholipid antibodies *CBC* *BMP* *UA*

(Continued)

Case	Diagnosis	HPI	PMH	PE Findings	Work Up
Middle age woman with joint pain, swelling of the hands, low grade fever, and fatigue for several mos	Lyme	Erythema migrans rash Arthralgias/myalgias Onset: migratory polyarticular Progression: monoarticular Hx of tick bite Lives in Northeast, mid-Atlantic or upper Midwest		+ Bell's palsy + bradycardia + heart block (Target rash will not be present at this stage)	Lyme titer—ELISA/Western blot EKG
Middle aged woman with pain in left hip	Osteoarthritis	Morning stiffness <30 min Monoarticular/polyarticular Asymmetric Insidious progression Aggravated by exercise Relieved by rest	FH Obesity Trauma/repetitive stress Previous surgery	< ROM	Hip x-ray
Middle aged woman with pain in left hip	Polymyalgia Rheumatica	Morning stiffness >30 min (Proximal) Distal extremities Fatigue Anorexia/weight loss Fever Headaches Scalp tenderness	Carpal tunnel syndrome Temporal arteritis	PIP affected + nodules	ESR CRP MRI or U/S of involved joints temporal artery bx? r/o polymyositis
Middle aged woman with pain in left hip (CRAB)	Multiple Myeloma	Bone pain: spine, long bones, skull, pelvis, chest Severe/intermittent Aggravated by movement Relieved by rest Fatigue/generalized weakness Weight loss	Anemia Recent bacterial infections	+ Back pain	SPEP U/A Bence Johns Proteins&Alb Peripheral smear Skeletal survey Serum Ca Cr CBC - anemia

(Continued)

Case	Diagnosis	HPI	PMH	PE Findings	Work Up
Patient complains of pain in left foot	**Gout**	Acute onset Swelling of ankle joint Monoarticular or oligoarticular Asymmetric Increased from foods with purines Increased with exercise Low grade fever	Prior episode Trauma/diuretics Alcohol/ nephrolithiasis metabolic syndrome	+ podagra + erythema	Joint aspiration with synovial fluid analysis x-ray of ankle
Patient complains of pain in left lower leg	**Peripheral artery disease**	Occurs with ambulation Occurs with climbing stairs Alleviated when exertion stops Intermittent/ cramping	Hyperlipidemia/ DM/MI/ HTA/smoker/+ FHx	+ diminished/ absent pulses + shiny skin/ absent hair + cold feet + thickened toe nails impaired Motor/sensation/ reflexes	Ankle/brachial arterial pressure Index (ABI) Duplex U/S
Patient complains of pain in left lower leg	**Cellulitis**	Ankle area extending up LLE +/- puncture wound Swelling/erythema/ unilateral Fever/chills/malaise No drainage	Trauma few days prior Skin disorder at site DM/HIV Surgery	+ lymph nodes + erythema	CBC w/ diff
Pediatric case with mother who complains of child becoming irritable lately	**Lead poisoning**	Anorexia (picky eater) Abdominal pain/ constipation Poor attention span Distractibility Impulsiveness/ hyperactivity Pica/lethargy Vomiting/headache	Lives in old building Low socioeconomic status		Physical Exam Blood Lead Level CBC

(Continued)

Case	Diagnosis	HPI	PMH	PE Findings	Work Up
Pediatric case with mother who complains of child becoming irritable lately	**Iron deficiency anemia**	Anorexia (picky eater) Lethargy Fatigue Pallor Irritability Poor feeding PICA Diet mainly of milk	Low birth weight Blood loss Systolic murmur		Physical exam Peripheral smear Serum iron/ ferritin TIBC/FEP Reticulocyte count FOB CBC/MCV/RDW
Pediatric case with mother who complains of child becoming irritable lately	**Attention Deficit Hyperactivity Disorder**	Inattention/ hyperactivity Impulsivity/ + Multiple settings Onset prior to age 12 Duration at least 6 mos Distracted/ disorganized Forgetful Constant fidgeting Short attention span Tasks not completed	FH + psychiatric disorders		Physical examination Psychiatric mental status evaluation
Patient complains of fatigue	**Hypothyroidism**	Weight (gain) Cold intolerance/dry skin Brittle hair/puffy face/ sleepiness Constipation/ depressed mood Muscle weakness Decreased sweating/ hoarseness Lower extremity edema Impaired memory Tongue enlargement	Potential drug-induced–Li Hypothalamic-pituitary axis damage Menstrual abnormalities Carpal tunnel syndrome History of autoimmune disease FH of hypothyroidism	+ loss of eye brows/periorbital edema + thyroid + deep tendon reflexes delayed relaxation + edema	TSH Free T4

(Continued)

Case	Diagnosis	HPI	PMH	PE Findings	Work Up
Patient complains of fatigue	B 12 deficiency	Weight loss Decreased appetite Unsteady gait Numbness/tingling of feet and hands Perception of wearing stocking or glove Constipation or diarrhea Sore tongue/ weakness Psychosis/memory loss Pallor Palpitations/DOE	Vegan diet Alcoholic Pernicious anemia– Crohn's disease/ celiac sprue GI resection Acid-suppressing drugs Metformin Bacterial overgrowth	Extremities–MRS + Romberg + Altered gait	CBC Serum B12 level Methylmalonic acid/ homocysteine level Peripheral smear
Patient complains of fatigue	Iron deficiency anemia	Angular cheilitis PICA Lethargy/pallor Palpitations/DOE Poor exercise tolerance Lightheadedness/leg cramps Glossitis/koilonychia	GI bleed/ menorrhagia/ celiac sprue Recent infections Bacterial overgrowth Systolic murmur	Pallor Tachycardia	Peripheral smear Serum iron/ ferritin TIBC/CBC
Vaginal discharge	**Bacterial Vaginosis**	Grayish white thin watery discharge Malodorous Post-menstrual onset	IUD Douching practice Recent antibiotics Menopause		Pelvic exam Wet /saline prep Vaginal pH Whiff test
Vaginal discharge	**Trichimonis Vaginitis**	Copious green– yellow frothy discharge Malodorous Pruritic Dyspareunia Dysuria Post-coital bleeding	Unprotected intercourse Multiple sexual partners IUD/smoker		Pelvic exam Wet / saline prep Vaginal pH

(Continued)

Case	Diagnosis	HPI	PMH	PE Findings	Work Up
Vaginal discharge	**Candida Vaginitis**	White thick cheesy discharge Odorless Pruritic Dyspareunia Dysuria	Previous episodes Recent antibiotics Diabetes/ pregnancy HIV/OCP		Pelvic exam KOH prep Vaginal pH
Vaginal discharge	**Atrophic Vaginitis**	Vaginal dryness Dysuria/urgency/ frequency Hot flashes Post-coital bleeding	Sleep disturbances Osteoporosis Pelvic organ prolapse Tamoxifen/lupron Menopause		Pelvic exam FSH → F/u menopause Estradiol Vaginal smear
53 y/o male c/o recurrent chest pain, dyspnea, and anxiety	**MI**	Diaphoresis Crushing pain >20 min Location: chest, neck, lower jaw, and down left arm FHx of heart disease SOB	Smoker Previous Hx of angina or MI	Tachycardia Hemodynamic instability	EKG/CK-MB Troponins
53 y/o male c/o recurrent chest pain, dyspnea, and anxiety	**Angina**	Pain <20 min Gradual onset Quality: discomfort rather than pain/ pressure/heaviness/ tightness/ constriction Location: center or left of chest Aggravated by exertion Alleviate by rest No change with respiration or position SOB	Previous Hx of angina Previous Hx of high cholesterol Previous Hx of HBP	Levine sign High blood pressure S3 or S4	EKG exercise Stress test

(Continued)

Case	Diagnosis	HPI	PMH	PE findings	Work up
53 y/o male c/o recurrent chest pain, dyspnea, and anxiety	GERD	Postprandial discomfort Aggravated by lying down Heartburn Regurgitation Dysphagia Chest pain Nausea		Wheezing	Esophageal PH monitoring EGD
Middle age male with severe chest pain	Aortic Dissection	"Tearing" chest pain Back pain Acute onset	Cocaine Hx of HBP	Hypertension BP asymmetry on UE UE pulselessness Hemodynamic instability	CXR Transesophageal echo CT scan *angio* U/Tox
Middle age male with severe chest pain	Cocaine-induced ACS	Chest pain Agitation	Cocaine Myocarditis Vasculitis	Hypertension Arrhythmias Nasal septum perforation	EKG /CK-MB Troponins I/T U/ToX
Middle age male with severe chest pain	PE	SOB/orthopnea acute onset Pleuritic pain Dyspnea at rest or with exertion (73%) Cough Calf or thigh pain and/or swelling hemoptysis	Smoking Hx of immobilization or recent flight	Hypertension/ hypothension Tachypnea Tachycardia Wheezing Calf or thigh swelling	VQScan Helical CT (ABG) *Lower ext duplex V/S*
67 y/o female with significant dyspneea and swelling of the legs in the past several weeks	CHF/Pulmonary Edema	SOB PND Orthopnea Cough (pink frothy sputum) Non-compliant with medication	HBP MI	JVD Peripheral edema Lung rales at the base	ECG/ECO BNP/Troponins CXR *lytes*

(Continued)

Case	Diagnosis	HPI	PMH	PE findings	Work up
67 y/o female with significant dyspneea and swelling of the legs in the past several weeks	Myocarditis	Chest pain Fatigue	Hx of URI		ECG/ECO BNP/Troponins CXR
67 y/o female with significant dyspnea and swelling of the legs in past several weeks	Arrhythmias (Atrial Fibrillation)	Palpitations Irregularly irregular pulse Lightheadedness Anxiety			ECG Holter 24-48 h Event recorder *w/u cause TSH BNP*
67 y/o female with significant dyspneea and swelling of the legs in past several weeks	Cor pulmonale/ COPD	SOB on exertion Exertional syncope Exertional angina	Hx of lung disease	S3/S4 Split S2	CXR ECG Ecocardiography
60 y/o male complaining of chest pain and cough	Pneumonia	Cough SOB Purulent sputum Chest pain	Recent viral prodrome	Febrile Mild respiratory distress Tachypnea Crackles Areas of lung consolidation	CXR Blood culture Sputum gram stain & culture CBC w/ differential
60 y/o male complaining of chest pain and cough	Pleural Effusion	Chest pain Aggravated by deep breath or motion Cough SOB	Recent viral prodrome	Febrile Mild respiratory distress Dullness Egophony	CXR Chest U/S Pleural fluid cell count/ cytology/ histology/ culture LDH/pH Sputum culture
60 y/o male complaining of chest pain and cough	Pericarditis	Sharp pleuritic chest pain Alleviated by position change (leaning forward or sitting) Persistent fever	Recent viral prodrome	Febrile Mild respiratory distress Pericardial friction rub Rash on the skin	ECG Echocardiogram CXR Blood cultures

(Continued)

Case	Diagnosis	HPI	PMH	PE findings	Work up
Elderly men with worsening dyspneea of exertion and productive cough	Chronic asthma	SOB early in life Sx aggravated at night/early morning	Hx of allergies Hx of smoking Exposure to second-hand smoke	Tachypneea Prolonged expirations Diffuse wheezing Increased vocal fremitus Intercostal retractions	PFTs Methacholine chalange
Elderly men with worsening dyspneea of exertion and productive cough	COPD	SOB in mid-life Slowly progressive Morning white sputum	Hx of smoking Hx of lung disease	Tachypneea Prolonged expirations Distant breath sounds Barrel chest	PFTs Chest CT CXR Pulse oximetry ABG
Elderly men with worsening dyspneea of exertion and productive cough	TB	Productive cough Weight loss Night sweats Previous TB contact	Hx of smoking HIV Immunossuppressed	Fever Tachypneea Cachexia	PPD IGRA CXR
Elderly men with worsening dyspneea of exertion and productive cough	Central airway obstruction (Bronchogenic carcinoma)	Cough Slowly progressive dyspnea Weight loss hemoptysis	Hx of smoking	Tachypneea Prolonged expirations Wheezing	Chest CT Bronchoscopy CXR
Middle age man with acute shortens of breath and agitation	Primary Spontaneous Pneumothorax	SOB Sudden onset Pleuritic chest pain Male Thin	Previous episodes of spontaneous pneumothorax	Tachypnea Decreased chest excursion on the affected side Diminished breath sounds Hyperresonance	CXR CT chest
Middle aged man with acute shortens of breath and agitation	COPD Exacerbation	Acute SOB exacerbation Productive cough Fatigue	Hx of lung disease Hx of smoking	Tachypnea Decreased chest excursion Barrel chest Hyperresonance	CXR ECG Ecocardiography

(Continued)

Case	Diagnosis	HPI	PMH	PE findings	Work up
41 y/o female in acute painful abdominal distress; the pain is persistent and she appears ill and very uncomfortable	PUD	Epigastric pain Epigastric fullness Nausea/vomiting Hematemeisis Melena	Hx of NSAIDs Hx of previous *H. Pilori*	Epigastrictenderness	Endoscopy FOB
41 y/o female in acute painful abdominal distress; the pain is persistent and she appears ill and very uncomfortable	Pancreatitis	Severe epigastric pain Radiates to the back Relieved by sitting up or bending forward Nausea/vomiting	Hx of alcohol Hx of gallstones	Epigastrictenderness Rebound Guarding Cullen/Grey Turner sign Febrile Tachycardic	Serum Amilase/Lipase Trypsinogen activation peptide CRP/ALT/AST *Bilirubi* Abd/CXR Abd U/S Abd CT ~~Hct~~ BUN
41 y/o female in acute painful abdominal distress; the pain is persistent and she appears ill and very uncomfortable	Acute cholecystitis	RUQ /EPIG pain radiates to right shoulder or back Nausea/vomiting	Multiple pregnancies Obeze	Murphy sign Febrile Tachycardic	CBC w dif. Abd U/S HIDA scan if U/S nl
68 y/o female with chills, nausea, and abdominal pain; she is frail and appears in mild discomfort	Hepatitis A	Fatigue Malaise Anorexia Nausea/vomiting, gradual onset	Sick contacts	Fever RUQ pain Hepato-splenomegaly Jaundice LAD	AST/ALT Bilirubin AlkP/GGT LDH Serum Ig M/Ig G Anti-HAV *IgM IgG Anti HAV*
68 y/o female with chills, nausea and abdominal pain; she is frail and appears in mild discomfort	Gastroenteritis	Diarrhea Vomiting/nausea Abd pain Onset in winter season		Fever Diffuse tenderness Dehydration	Blood Culture FOB Fecal leukocyte Fecal lactoferrin *indicates inflammation*

(Continued)

Case	Diagnosis	HPI	PMH	PE findings	Work up
68 y/o female with chills, nausea, and abdominal pain; she is frail and appears in mild discomfort	Acute cholangitis	Abdominal pain Jaundice Nausea/Vomiting		Fever RUQ pain	CBC w dif/CRP ALT/AST/GGT/ Alk Phosphatase Blood cultures Transabdominal U/S *ERCP*
Male with increasing abdominal pain and restless due to pain	Diverticulitis	Abd pain frequently localized in LLQ Duration several days Gradual increasing Diarrhea Constipation		Fever LLQ tenderness Guarding Rebound	CT scan Abd x-ray CBC w dif
Male with increasing abdominal pain and restless due to pain	Large bowel obstruction	Severe cramping abd pain Difuse & poorly localized Accentuated in waves Vomiting Constipation Unable to pass flatulus	Hx of prior abd. surgery	Fever Abd distention Increase peristalsis	CBC w/ differential Electrolytes/ anion gap Ba Enema Abd x-ray Colonoscopy Abd CT scan
Male with increasing abdominal pain and restless due to pain	Nephrolithiasis	Excruciating back & flank pain w/ rapid onset Radiating to groin or abdomen Nausea/vomiting Anorexia Dysuria	Hx of kidney stone	Fever CVA tenderness	Helical renal CT Hematuria U/A for Ca, Oxalates, Uric Acid
Young man c/o headache	Meningitis	Severe headache Photophobia Nuchal rigidity Feverish	Rash or recent URI Recent travel	+ Brudsinki Nuchal rigidity	CBC w/diff Serum glucose electrolytes Blood c/s x3 CT head LP

(Continued)

Case	Diagnosis	HPI	PMH	PE findings	Work up
Middle aged man c/o headache	**Subarachnoid hemorrhage**	Photophobia Nuchal rigidity Sudden onset LOC Confusion Vomiting	Recent h/o head injury	Nuchal rigidity MMSE altered	CT head
Young woman c/o headache	**Migraine**	Unilateral headache Pulsating in nature Photophobia Visual disturbance A/w food, menses Nausea Precipitated by stress, hunger, and fatigue	OCP use FH of similar headaches		*Clinical Dx*
Patient c/o dizziness	**Panic Attack**	+ dizziness occurs during recurrent, unexpected episodes of panic attacks + persistent concern about future attacks Attacks w sweating, trembling, SOB, CP, palpitations, and circumoral numbness	+ h/o anxiety No h/o substance abuse FH + caffeine use		*MSE*
Patient c/o dizziness	**Alcohol Intoxication**	+ dizziness + euphoria + ataxia + slurred speech + vomiting + confusion	h/o alcohol abuse + FH of alcoholism + Stressful job	Alcohol scent on breathe Gait unstable Slurred speech MMSE	Serum ethanol level Urine toxicology Serum glucose level *+/- thiamine*

(Continued)

Blood sugar utox Serum ethanol

Case	Diagnosis	HPI	PMH	PE findings	Work up
65 yo man c/o forgetfulness	Alzheimer's Disease	Older patient + progressive memory loss + progressive difficulty with ADL	FH	MMSE	MRI brain PET brain
23 yo man c/o restlessness	Schizophrenia	At least 6 mo h/o delusions, hallucinations (auditory), social dysfunction, and disorganized speech	FH	MMSE + impaired judgment	Urine tox screen CT of head MRI of brain PET brain
18 yo man c/o restlessness	Attention Deficit Hyperactivity Disorder	+ At least 6 mo h/o inattentiveness, hyperactivity, and impulsivity + interferes with functioning + symptoms present in multiple settings	FH	MMSE	Urine toxicology
55 yo woman c/o urinary incontinence	Urge incontinence	Obese Urinary urgency No precipitating factors but can be precipitated by cold weather or sound of running water	+ h/o UTI + h/o DM + h/o BPH (men) Surgeries: C-section (women), prostate (men) Pregnancy/delivery	No tenderness No CVAT	Genital and pelvic exams UA Cystometry Post void residual volume Pelvic or abdominal U/S

(Continued)

Case	Diagnosis	HPI	PMH	PE findings	Work up
55 yo woman c/o urinary incontinence	Stress incontinence	Post-menopausal Obese Leakage with coughing, laughing, sneezing or exercising Denies urinary urgency	+ h/o constipation + h/o urinary incontinence + Multiple pregnancies/deliveries + h/o smoking + h/o prostatectomy (in men)	No tenderness No CVAT	Genital and pelvic exams UA Cystometry Post void residual volume Pelvic or abdominal U/S
37 yo woman with flank pain	Pyelonephritis	+ Dysuria + Feverish + Nausea and vomiting + Urinary frequency + Urinary urgency + Hematuria + Chills	+ h/o recurrent UTI + h/o BPH (men)	Fever + CVAT	U/A *CBC* Urine culture Renal U/S *CT if not responding to Tx*
37 yo woman with flank pain	Nephrolithiasis	+ Intermittent pain + Radiates to groin + Hematuria + Urinary urgency	FH + h/o dehydration + Diet high in protein and sodium + Overweight	Afebrile + CVAT	U/A Renal U/S CT abd
37 yo man with groin pain	Testicular torsion	Young adolescent men Sudden severe testicular pain Unilateral Pain radiates to lower back Nausea and vomiting			Genital exam Doppler U/S of scrotum

(Continued)

Case	Diagnosis	HPI	PMH	PE findings	Work up
63 yo man c/o vertigo	**Benign Positional Vertigo**	Older patient + episodic, each lasting a few min + loss of balance during episodes + N/V + sudden onset Precipitated by change in head position Denies weakness and numbness Denies slurred speech			Dix-Hallpike test CBC w/diff ╱ CT of head ╱ Audiogram ╱
65 yo man c/o vertigo	**Cerebrovascular accident**	+ focal neuro deficits + symptoms lasting >2 hrs + sudden onset	h/o HTN h/o DM h/o high blood cholesterol h/o atrial fibrillation Not compliant with warfarin FH of early CAD + Smoking history	Focal neurological deficits	Cholesterol, HDL, LDL, triglycerides CT head Doppler U/S of carotids EKG *echo*
45 yo woman with muscle weakness	**Myasthenia gravis**	Weakness worse at night and with exertion Weakness alleviated with rest + diplopia + difficulty chewing and swallowing + Slurred speech + droopy eyelids + progressive fatigue + jaw weakness with chewing + difficulty walking up stairs Denies muscle pain	FH of hypothyroidism and RA	Slurred speech Drooping eyelids Decreased muscle strength decreased reflexes in UE and LE b/l	Acetylcholine receptor antibodies Muscle specific tyrosine kinase antibodies Anti-striated muscle antibodies (anti-SM) EMG, NCS *anti-ach* *anti TMSTK* *anti SM* *(mg/NCS*

(Continued)

Case	Diagnosis	HPI	PMH	PE findings	Work up
45 yo man with muscle weakness	**Guillan-Barre Syndrome**	+ ascending symmetrical weakness + numbness and tingling + progressive fatigue + diplopia + slurred speech Denies urinary incontinence	Recent URI	Low BP and high HR Eyes: + ptosis Loss of deep tendon reflexes in LE b/l Decreased muscle strength in LE b/l	EMG, NCS FVC, negative inspiratory force (NIF)
50 yo man c/o bloody stools	**Colon Cancer**	+ painless rectal bleeding + unintentional weight loss + constipation + change in stool caliber + high red meat diet + fatigue	No screening colonoscopy + h/o anemia FH of colon cancer + Smoking history		Rectal exam with FOB CBC w/diff CT abdomen Colonoscopy
60 yo man c/o bloody stools	**Angiodysplasia**	+ painless rectal bleeding + stool black and tarry + no recent weight loss + fatigue No weight loss No h/o easy bruising	+ h/o anemia No FH of colon cancer ↓ *wju melims*		Rectal exam with FOB CBC w/diff PT, PTT, INR *Cing* CT abdomen Colonoscopy EGD
40 yo man c/o bloody stools	**Diverticulosis**	+ painless rectal bleeding + constipation + feeling of weakness + dizziness + low fiber diet + low fluid intake No weight loss	No fiber supplements + h/o HTN + h/o IBS FH of diverticulosis No family h/o colon cancer		Rectal exam with FOB CBC w/ diff Abdominal x-ray Abdominal CT Colonoscopy

Putting it All Together

Putting It All Together: CIS, SEP, and ICE

8

The following 31 cases are designed to give you additional practice with Step 2 CS–style scenarios. They should be used after you have reviewed all of the earlier chapters in this book. Remember, when you take the CS exam, you'll need to pass all 3 components in order to get an overall passing score.

Depending on your individual strengths and weaknesses, you can select how to best use these cases to your advantage.

Option 1: If you need practice on all 3 components: CIS, SEP, and ICE

Practice these cases with a study partner. Play the "role" of the doctor (don't read the case before your study session).

- Your study partner will play the role of the patient (he/she will need to review the case prior to the study session to answer the questions appropriately).
- Set a timer for 15 minutes before you start.
- Read the "doorway information" and write down the necessary information on a scrap sheet of paper (mnemonics and a differential diagnosis for the chief complaint).
- Knock on the door, introduce yourself, and start on the focused history/focused physical exam on the "patient" (your study partner).
- Assess your ability to identify the CIS sub-components using the checklist for the case.
- If English is not your first language, practice the common phrases reviewed in this book.
- Your study partner can also mark the information you are able to elicit from the history. Review the checklist afterward and think about what questions you should have asked. Remember, there is no history checklist on the exam; this is simply a tool to assist your preparation for the exam.
- The physical exam checklist provides a suggested focused physical exam for each case. Your study partner should share with you as many of the findings as possible.

After the 15 minutes is over, reset your timer for 10 minutes and type a Patient Note. **Use the Patient Note template** available at **usmle.org/practice-materials**. The most efficient way to improve your Patient Notes is to practice using the USMLE template, and type lots and lots of notes!

After completing the above steps, grade your own Patient Notes using the provided samples. Have your study partner grade CIS, SEP, and the physical examination components of ICE using the appropriate checklists.

Option 2: If you need practice only with writing the Patient Note

As you review each case, use the margins as you would use scrap paper on the exam to write down any important findings.

- Begin to draw a mental picture of the patient and the differential diagnosis.
- Predict what you think the relevant history and physical exam items would be.
- Type a Patient Note using the USMLE template, including the significant positives and negatives from the history and physical exam.
- Indicate your list of differential diagnoses with justifications and diagnostic workup plans.

Review your predictions and notes with the answers found in the **patient notes** that follow.

CASE 1: FATIGUE, COUGH, AND CHEST PAIN

(handwritten notes in right margin):
DDx
lung cancer   TB   Pneumonia
COPD + exacerbation
PNA
ACS

Doorway Information

Opening Scenario

Daniel Johnson, a 52-year-old man, presents with fatigue and cough for the past 6 months, and chest pain for the past 2 days.

Vital Signs

T 38.2 C (100.8 F)

BP 132/90 mm Hg

Pulse 91/min

Respirations 22/min

Pulse oximetry 92% on room air

Examinee Tasks

1. Obtain a focused history.

2. Perform a relevant physical exam. Do not perform rectal, pelvic, genitourinary, or corneal reflex exam.

3. Discuss your initial diagnostic impression and your workup plan with the patient.

4. After leaving the room, complete your Patient Note.

Communication and Interpersonal Skills Checklist

Fostering the Relationship	Gathering Information	Providing Information
☐ Knocked	☐ Elicited chief complaint	☐ Summarized significant information
☐ Introduced self	☐ Established timeline of patient's CC (chief complaint)	☐ Provided diagnostic impression
☐ Clarified role	☐ Used open-ended question	☐ Justified diagnosis with evidence from encounter
☐ Was properly groomed	☐ Used non-leading questions	☐ Assessed patient's need for additional information
☐ Made eye contact	☐ Used closed-ended questions	☐ Encouraged and answered questions
☐ Maintained appropriate distance	☐ Asked one question at a time	☐ Assessed patient's comprehension of probable illness
☐ Displayed confident manner	☐ Did not use medical jargon	
☐ Showed care and concern	☐ Appropriately used "continuers"	
☐ Was respectful and nonjudgmental	☐ Paraphrased	
☐ Established patient's preferred title	☐ Appropriately used transitions	
☐ Used proper draping	☐ Elicited additional concerns	
☐ Focused on patient	☐ Assessed impact on patient's life	
☐ Did not interrupt patient	☐ Checked for patient understanding	
☐ Maintained appropriate and responsive body language		

Making Decisions	Supporting Emotions
☐ Clearly stated next steps in management	☐ Actively listened and validated patient's expectations
☐ **Counseled** patient	☐ Showed empathy and used appropriate reassurances
☐ Agreed to **mutual plan** of action	☐ Inquired about patient's support system
	☐ Managed the **challenge** (here; patient asked, "Is it serious?")

History and Physical Examination Checklist

HPI

- ☐ Worsening cough
  - ☐ Duration: 6 Months
- ☐ dry and hacking
- ☐ Sputum
  - ☐ Blood tinged
  - ☐ Rusty colored
  - ☐ Small quantity
- ☐ Night sweats
- ☐ Low grade fever
- ☐ Chest pain
  - ☐ Right sided
  - ☐ Sharp
  - ☐ Worse when he breaths deeply
  - ☐ Started a few days ago
  - ☐ Pain 4/10
  - ☐ No radiation
- ☐ Improves with cough suppressants and OTC acetaminophen
- ☐ No orthopnea
- ☐ No SOB
- ☐ 20 lb weight loss
  - ☐ Over the last 4 months
  - ☐ Doesn't feel hungry

PMH

- ☐ No similar illness
- ☐ History of previous recurrent pneumonia
  - ☐ Treated
  - ☐ Did not make follow up visits
- ☐ No hospitalizations or surgery
- ☐ Meds: no prescription meds
- ☐ OTC: acetaminophen
- ☐ NKDA

Family Hx

- ☐ No significant family history
- ☐ Not been around anyone sick recently

Social Hx

- ☐ Recently released from prison
- ☐ Longtime cellmate with serious cough
- ☐ History of sex with men
- ☐ Unsure of HIV status
- ☐ Heroin use
- ☐ Smokes 1–2 packs per day
- ☐ No alcohol use

Physical Examination

- ☐ Washed hands prior to examination
- ☐ Inspected orophayrnx
- ☐ Palpated neck/axilla for lymphadenopathy
- ☐ Palpated chest for tactile fremitus
  - ☐ tactile fremitus bilaterally
- ☐ Palpated chest wall for tenderness
- ☐ Percussed lungs posteriorly bilaterally
- ☐ Percussed lungs anteriorly bilaterally
- ☐ Ausculated lungs posteriorly bilaterally
  - ☐ few bibasilar rales
- ☐ Aucultated lungs anteriorly bilaterally
  - ☐ few bibasilar rales
- ☐ Auscultated heart (4 areas: A, P, T, M)
- ☐ Examined extremities for clubbing, cyanosis, and/or edema

Patient Note

History

HPI: 52 y/o man presents with cough and fatigue for the past 6 mos. The cough has been getting progressively worse, and is associated with occasional small amount of blood tinged sputum (rusty-colored). He also complains of fatigue, night sweats and low grade fevers. Over last 2 days he has been experiencing sharp, pleuritic right sided chest pain (4/10) that does not radiate. He denies orthopnea and acute SOB. He admits to 20 lb weight loss over past 4 mos and loss of appetite, He also reports having had several episodes of "pneumonia." He is sexually active with men and his HIV status is unknown. He has been taking occasional acetaminophen and OTC cough suppressants for his symptoms. He smokes 1-2 packs of cigarettes per day and was recently released from prison.

Physical Examination

T 100.8 F, respirations 22/min, pulse 91/min, BP 132/90 mm Hg

Pulse oximetry 92% on room air

General: In moderate respiratory distress, but cooperative

HEENT: Oropharynx - no erythema, exudates, ulcers or thrush.

Chest: Bibasilar rales and decreased tactile fremitus bilaterally

Cough on expiration, pleuritic pain on right with deep inspiration

CV: Sl/S2 WNL, RRR, no M/R/G

Ext: no edema, clubbing or cyanosis

Data Interpretation

DIAGNOSIS 1. PULMONARY TUBERCULOSIS

History Findings	Physical Exam Findings
6 month cough	Fever and tachypnea
Blood tinged sputum	Moderate respiratory distress
Night sweats	Pleuritic pain on right
Low-grade fever	Cough on expiration
Fatigue	Rales and decreased tactile fremitus bilaterally
Sharp, pleuritic right-sided chest pain	
20 lb weight loss over past 4 mos	
Recent prison release	

DIAGNOSIS 2. PNEUMOCYSTIS JIROVECI PNEUMONIA

History Findings	Physical Exam Findings
6 month cough	Fever and tachypnea
Blood tinged sputum	Moderate respiratory distress
Low-grade fever	Pleuritic pain on right
History of sex with men	
Unknown HIV status	
Sharp, pleuritic right-sided chest pain	
Weight loss	

Diagnostic Studies

CBC w/differential

CXR PA and lateral

Sputum for gram stain and culture

PPD with controls   IGRA

HIV RNA PCR

Handwritten margin notes:
labs
imaging
micro
path

- CBC w/ dif
- HIV PCR
- IGRA
- CT chest
sputum gs/clx

CASE 2: BACK PAIN AND FEVER

Doorway Information

Opening Scenario

Jane Williams is a 63-year-old woman who presents with back pain and fever for the past 3 days.

[handwritten: circle around "63-year-"]

Vital Signs

T 38.3 C (101.0 F) *[handwritten: Febrile]*

BP 129/85 mm Hg

Pulse 108/min *[handwritten: tachy]*

Respirations 16/min

Examinee Tasks

1. Obtain a focused history.

2. Perform a relevant physical exam. Do not perform rectal, pelvic, genitourinary, female breast, or corneal reflex exam.

3. Discuss your initial diagnostic impression and your workup plan with the patient. *[handwritten: lung, back, LE neuro, abdominal exam]*

4. After leaving the room, complete your patient note.

Communication and Interpersonal Skills Checklist

Fostering the Relationship	Gathering Information	Providing Information
☐ Knocked	☐ Elicited chief complaint	☐ Summarized significant information
☐ Introduced self	☐ Established timeline of patient's CC (chief complaint)	☐ Provided diagnostic impression
☐ Clarified role	☐ Used open-ended question	☐ Justified diagnosis with evidence from encounter
☐ Was properly groomed	☐ Used non-leading questions	☐ Assessed patient's need for additional information
☐ Made eye contact	☐ Used closed-ended questions	☐ Encouraged and answered questions
☐ Maintained appropriate distance	☐ Asked one question at a time	☐ Assessed patient's comprehension of probable illness
☐ Displayed confident manner	☐ Did not use medical jargon	
☐ Showed care and concern	☐ Appropriately used "continuers"	
☐ Was respectful and nonjudgmental	☐ Paraphrased	
☐ Established patient's preferred title	☐ Appropriately used transitions	
☐ Used proper draping	☐ Elicited additional concerns	
☐ Focused on patient	☐ Assessed impact on patient's life	
☐ Did not interrupt patient	☐ Checked for patient understanding	
☐ Maintained appropriate and responsive body language		

Making Decisions	Supporting Emotions
☐ Clearly stated next steps in management	☐ Actively listened and validated patient's expectations
☐ **Counseled** patient	☐ Showed empathy and used appropriate reassurances
☐ Agreed to **mutual plan** of action	☐ Inquired about patient's support system
	☐ Managed the **challenge** (here; patient asked, "Can I have something for the pain?")

History and Physical Examination Checklist

HPI

- ☐ Nausea and fatigue
- ☐ Duration: 3 days
- ☐ Patient assumed it was flu initially
- ☐ Progressively felt worse
- ☐ Back pain
  - ☐ Dull
  - ☐ 5/10 intensity
  - ☐ Constant
  - ☐ Radiates to groin
- ☐ Increased urinary frequency
- ☐ + burning during urination
- ☐ No blood in urine or discoloration
- ☐ + fever
- ☐ + chills
- ☐ Fever alleviated by Acetaminophen
- ☐ No other aggravating or alleviating factors

PMH

- ☐ Recurrent urinary tract infections
- ☐ Last episode 1 year ago
- ☐ No history of kidney stones
- ☐ History of diabetes mellitus type 2
- ☐ Diabetic foot ulcer
- ☐ Recent HgA1c 6.8%
- ☐ HTN
- ☐ Meds: metformin and lisinopril
- ☐ NKDA

Family Hx

- ☐ No relevant family history

Social Hx

- ☐ No alcohol, no drugs
- ☐ No tobacco use

Physical Examination

- ☐ Washed hands prior to examination
- ☐ Inspected abdomen
- ☐ Auscultated abdomen in 4 quadrants
- ☐ Percussed abdomen in 4 quadrants
- ☐ Palpated abdomen in 4 quadrants
- ☐ Checked for rebound tenderness
- ☐ Examined for costovertebral angle tenderness (CVAT)
  - ☐ Positive
- ☐ Palpated lumbar spine and paraspinal muscles
- ☐ Performed straight leg raise test
- ☐ Examined extremities
  - ☐ Ulceration on plantar surface

Patient Note

History

HPI: 63 y/o woman presents with right sided pain of her mid to lower back and fever for 3 days. Has nausea and fatigue. She thought she had the flu and stayed in bed with plenty of fluids and rest. 1 day later the chills and fever started. She describes the pain as dull and constant, with radiation to the groin. Pain is 5/10. Acetaminophen reduced fever only. She c/o burning pain during urination and increased frequency but denies any blood in urine. No vomiting, diarrhea, constipation, numbness and tingling, chest pain or headache.

PMH: HTN and type 2 DM. Previous hx of recurrent UTI (last episode 1 yr ago). LMP 11 yrs ago; last Pap smear 3 yrs ago; G2P2

Medications: acetaminophen, metformin, and lisinopril. No recent dose changes. NKDA.

FH: not significant

SH: retired teacher, sexually active with husband of 42 yrs

No EtOH, tobacco, or drugs; no recent travel history

Physical Examination

T 38.3 C, BP 129/85 mm Hg, pulse 108/min, respirations 16/min

General: patient appears to be in mild discomfort due to pain, AAO x 3

Abd: no skin abnormalities, +BS x 4Q, tympanic x 4Q, suprapubic/RLQ tenderness, and CVA tenderness, rebound tenderness

Foot exam: ulcer on plantar surface of left small toe, partially healed

Neuro: negative straight leg raise

Data Interpretation

DIAGNOSIS 1. PYELONEPHRITIS

History Findings	Physical Exam Findings
Back pain	Suprapubic tenderness No rebound
History of fever, dysuria, chills, fatigue	Fever, tachycardia
Nausea	CVA tenderness

DIAGNOSIS 2. CYSTITIS

History Findings	Physical Exam Findings
Dysuria	Fever
↑ frequency	Suprapubic tenderness
Previous UTI	
Diabetes	

DIAGNOSIS 3. NEPHROLITHIASIS

History Findings	Physical Exam Findings
Back pain	Tenderness on palpation, suprapubic & RLQ
Radiation to groin	CVA tenderness
Nausea	Tachycardia
↑ frequency	
Dysuria	

Diagnostic Studies

CBC with differential

Urinalysis

Urine culture

CT abdomen/pelvis without IV contrast

CASE 3: BLOODY STOOLS

Doorway Information

Opening Scenario

Maria Mitchell is a 72-year-old woman who comes to the ER with a history of bloody stool for the past 1 day.

Vital Signs

T 36.7 C (98.0 F)

BP 108/55 mm Hg

Pulse 100/min

Respirations 12/min

Examinee Tasks

1. Obtain a focused history.

2. Perform a relevant physical exam. Do not perform rectal, pelvic, genitourinary, female breast, or corneal reflex exam.

3. Discuss your initial diagnostic impression and your workup plan with the patient.

4. After leaving the room, complete your patient note on the given form.

Communication and Interpersonal Skills Checklist		
Fostering the Relationship	**Gathering Information**	**Providing Information**
☐ Knocked ☐ Introduced self ☐ Clarified role ☐ Was properly groomed ☐ Made eye contact ☐ Maintained appropriate distance ☐ Displayed confident manner ☐ Showed care and concern ☐ Was respectful and nonjudgmental ☐ Established patient's preferred title ☐ Used proper draping ☐ Focused on patient ☐ Did not interrupt patient ☐ Maintained appropriate and responsive body language	☐ Elicited chief complaint ☐ Established timeline of patient's CC (chief complaint) ☐ Used open-ended question ☐ Used non-leading questions ☐ Used closed-ended questions ☐ Asked one question at a time ☐ Did not use medical jargon ☐ Appropriately used "continuers" ☐ Paraphrased ☐ Appropriately used transitions ☐ Elicited additional concerns ☐ Assessed impact on patient's life ☐ Checked for patient understanding	☐ Summarized significant information ☐ Provided diagnostic impression ☐ Justified diagnosis with evidence from encounter ☐ Assessed patient's need for additional information ☐ Encouraged and answered questions ☐ Assessed patient's comprehension of probable illness
Making Decisions	**Supporting Emotions**	
☐ Clearly stated next steps in management ☐ **Counseled** patient ☐ Agreed to **mutual plan** of action	☐ Actively listened and validated patient's expectations ☐ Showed empathy and used appropriate reassurances ☐ Inquired about patient's support system ☐ Managed the **challenge** (here; patient asked, "Will I die?")	

History and Physical Examination Checklist

HPI
- ☐ Blood in stool
- ☐ Noticed it earlier in the afternoon
- ☐ 3 episodes since
  - ☐ Last episode 1 hr ago
  - ☐ Blood mixed with stool
- ☐ Also on toilet paper
- ☐ Quantity of blood is "a lot"
- ☐ No associated pain
- ☐ No cramping
- ☐ Feels weak and dizzy
  - ☐ When she stands up after going to the bathroom
- ☐ No fever
- ☐ No chills
- ☐ No nausea or vomiting
- ☐ No diarrhea
- ☐ No history of constipation
- ☐ No weight loss

PMH
- ☐ No similar episodes in the past
- ☐ HTN
- ☐ Osteoporosis
- ☐ Cholecystectomy at 40
- ☐ Meds: Hydrochlorothiazide, multi-vitamins and occasional acetaminophen
- ☐ No anti-inflammatory drugs
- ☐ No anti-coagulants
- ☐ NKDA
- ☐ No past colonoscopy

Family Hx
- ☐ Parent deceased from heart disease in their 80's
- ☐ No family history of colon cancer
- ☐ No family history of IBD

Social Hx
- ☐ No alcohol, no drugs
- ☐ No tobacco use

Physical Examination

- ☐ Washed hands prior to examination
- ☐ Inspected abdomen
- ☐ Auscultated abdomen in 4 quadrants
- ☐ Percussed abdomen in 4 quadrants
- ☐ Lightly palpated abdomen in 4 quadrants
- ☐ Deeply palpated abdomen in non-tender quadrants
- ☐ Checked for guarding
- ☐ Checked for rebound
- ☐ Auscultated heart: 4 cardiac areas
- ☐ Auscultated lungs
- ☐ Examined distal pulses bilaterally

PAm 4R FOSS
I
T
S

Patient Note

History

HPI: 72 y/o woman presents with painless rectal bleeding for the past 1 day. She had 4 bowel movements with bright red blood per rectum over the past 1 day. There is no pain, cramping, or melena associated with her bowel movements. She denies fever, chills, nausea, vomiting, weight loss, and any recent change in bowel habits. She complains of feeling "weak and dizzy" when she stands up after going to the bathroom. She has not experienced rectal bleeding in the past. She has never had a screening colonoscopy.

PMH: HTN, osteoporosis

PSH: Cholecystectomy

NKDA

Medications: HCTZ, MVI, acetaminophen PRN pain

FH: no colon cancer

SH: No EtOH/tob/drug use

Physical Examination

Vitals: T: 98.0, blood pressure 108/55, pulse 100/min, respirations 12/min

Gen: Well appearing. In no apparent distress

CV: Normal S1/S2 , RRR, no murmurs, rubs or gallops

Lungs: Clear to auscultation B/L, no wheezes, rales, rhonchi

Abd: Well healed surgical scar in RUQ, no other skin lesions; bowel sounds presents in 4 quadrants, tympanic to percussion in all quadrants, no palpable masses, soft, nontender and nondistended. No guarding or rebound tenderness

Data Interpretation

DIAGNOSIS 1. DIVERTICULOSIS

History Findings	Physical Exam Findings
Hematochezia	No apparent distress (NAD)
Multiple bowel movements	Afebrile
Feeling of weakness	No abdominal masses
Dizziness	
No family history of colon cancer	

Diagnosis 2. Hemorrhoids

History Findings	Physical Exam Findings
Hematochezia	No abdominal masses
Denies any abdominal pain	Afebrile
No weight loss	

Diagnosis 3. Colon Cancer

History Findings	Physical Exam Findings
Hematochezia	
No previous colonoscopy	
Age	

Diagnostic Studies

Digital rectal exam

CBC w/differential

PT/PTT/INR

CT scan of abd/pelvis

Colonoscopy once stable

CASE 4: CHEST PAIN

Doorway Information

Opening Scenario

Maryann Peters is a 48-year-old woman who presents with chest pain for the past 4 hours.

Vital Signs

T 37 C (98.6 F)

BP 128/58 mm Hg

Pulse 108/min — *tachy*

Respirations 26/min — *tachy*

Oxygen saturation 91% on room air — *hypot*

Examinee Tasks

1. Obtain a focused history.

2. Perform a relevant physical exam. Do not perform rectal, pelvic, genitourinary, female breast, or corneal reflex exam.

3. Discuss your initial diagnostic impression and your workup with the patient.

anxiety
PE
ACS
costochondritis
Pneumothorax
pericarditis

Communication and Interpersonal Skills Checklist		
Fostering the Relationship	**Gathering Information**	**Providing Information**
☐ Knocked ☐ Introduced self ☐ Clarified role ☐ Was properly groomed ☐ Made eye contact ☐ Maintained appropriate distance ☐ Displayed confident manner ☐ Showed care and concern ☐ Was respectful and nonjudgmental ☐ Established patient's preferred title ☐ Used proper draping ☐ Focused on patient ☐ Did not interrupt patient ☐ Maintained appropriate and responsive body language	☐ Elicited chief complaint ☐ Established timeline of patient's CC (chief complaint) ☐ Used open-ended question ☐ Used non-leading questions ☐ Used closed-ended questions ☐ Asked one question at a time ☐ Did not use medical jargon ☐ Appropriately used "continuers" ☐ Paraphrased ☐ Appropriately used transitions ☐ Elicited additional concerns ☐ Assessed impact on patient's life ☐ Checked for patient understanding	☐ Summarized significant information ☐ Provided diagnostic impression ☐ Justified diagnosis with evidence from encounter ☐ Assessed patient's need for additional information ☐ Encouraged and answered questions ☐ Assessed patient's comprehension of probable illness
Making Decisions	**Supporting Emotions**	
☐ Clearly stated next steps in management ☐ **Counseled** patient ☐ Agreed to **mutual plan** of action	☐ Actively listened and validated patient's expectations ☐ Showed empathy and used appropriate reassurances ☐ Inquired about patient's support system ☐ Managed the **challenge** (here; patient asked, "Am I having a heart attack?")	

History and Physical Examination Checklist

HPI

- ☐ Chest pain
  - ☐ Substernal
  - ☐ Sharp
  - ☐ 6/10 intensity
  - ☐ No radiation
- ☐ Duration: 4 hours
- ☐ Onset while waiting for her baggage at the airport
- ☐ Recent trip to Japan — long flight
- ☐ No diaphoresis
- ☐ No nausea
- ☐ SOB
  - ☐ Progressively worse
  - ☐ Breathing makes the pain worse ↗
- ☐ Symptoms not improved by rest or Ibuprofen
- ☐ No fever
- ☐ No chills
- ☐ No cough
- ☐ No sick contacts
- ☐ No leg pain

PMH

- ☐ No similar episodes in the past
- ☐ No GERD
- ☐ HTN
- ☐ Diet controlled–low Na
- ☐ Meds: no prescription meds
- ☐ NKDA
- ☐ G1P1
- ☐ No miscarriages
- ☐ + Contraceptive pills

Family Hx

- ☐ No family history of blood clots or miscarriages
- ☐ No family history of IBD

Social Hx

- ☐ Alcohol at social events
- ☐ No recreational drugs
- ☐ Smokes ½ pack/day
  - ☐ 28 years
  - ☐ Trying to quit
- ☐ Married
- ☐ Works as a photographer
- ☐ Is physically active

Physical Examination

- ☐ Washed hands prior to examination
- ☐ Inspection of chest
- ☐ Auscultated heart and carotids
- ☐ Palpated chest for tenderness, location of PMI
  - ☐ Pain not reproduced by palpation
  - ☐ Pain not positional
  - ☐ PMI is not displaced
- ☐ Checked carotids, peripheral pulses and JVP
- ☐ Examined extremities for edema, clubbing, cyanosis, calf tenderness, and palpable cord
- ☐ Assessed Homan's sign
  - ☐ Negative bilaterally
- ☐ Auscultated lungs
  - ☐ Breathing is painful
- ☐ Assessed chest expansion
- ☐ Assessed tactile fremitus
- ☐ Percussed lungs

Patient Note

History

HPI: 48 y/o woman presents with substernal chest pain for the past 4 hrs, described as constant and sharp, 6/10 in intensity and non-radiating. Patient thought that lifting heavy luggage upon her arrival from a trip to Japan precipitated the pain. She is experiencing pleuritic chest pain and progressive dyspnea. Ibuprofen provided no relief of pain. No diaphoresis, nausea, fever, chills, cough, sick contacts, leg swelling or leg pain is noted on examination.

PMH: no similar complaints, NKDA, diet-controlled HTN

Meds: Oral contraceptives

FHx: no similar symptoms, no major illnesses and no history of blood clots

SH: 14 pack yrs, trying to quit, no EtOH or illicit drugs

Physical Examination

BP 128/58 mm Hg, Pulse 108/min, respirations 26/min, and oxygen saturation 91% on room air

General: alert, conscious and coherent; anxious and uncomfortable in respiratory distress

CV: Sl and S2 normal; RRR; no m, v, g; PMI not displaced; no carotid bruits; no JVD

Lungs: pain with inspiration and use of accessory muscles; equal chest expansion bilaterally; CTAB; no rales, wheezes, rhonchi or rubs; non-tender on palpation; no dullness on percussion; tactile fremitus symmetric and normal

Extremities: peripheral pulses palpable and equal bilaterally, 2+; no clubbing, cyanosis or pedal edema; no lower extremities varicosities, tenderness or palpable cords; negative Homan's sign

Data Interpretation

DIAGNOSIS 1. PULMONARY EMBOLISM

History Findings	Physical Exam Findings
Substernal chest pain, constant, sharp and non-radiating	Tachypnea
Pleuritic chest pain	Tachycardia pulse 108/min
Acute onset of chest pain	Pain with inspiration
Prolonged travel	Use of accessory muscles
Shortness of breath	Decreased oxygen saturation
Oral contraceptive pills	
Smoking for 14 pack yrs	
Female age >35	

Risk factors (handwritten annotation)

Diagnosis 2. Acute myocardial infarction

History Findings	Physical Exam Findings
Substernal chest pain, constant, sharp	Tachypnea
Shortness of breath	Tachycardia
Acute onset of chest pain	Decreased oxygen saturation
Smoking for 14 pack yrs	
History of hypertension	

Diagnosis 3. Pneumonia

History Findings	Physical Exam Findings
Substernal chest pain, constant, sharp and non-radiating	Tachypnea
Pleuritic chest pain	Tachycardia
Shortness of breath	Pain with inspiration
Smoking for 14 pack yrs	Use of accessory muscles
	Decreased oxygen saturation

Diagnostic Studies

ABG — AB disturbances

D-dimer — no

CBC with diff

PTT/PT/INR — PE

EKG, chest x-ray — r/o ACS

Troponin/CK-MB — PE

VQ scan or spiral CT — PE

Doppler U/S of lower extremities — PE

- trops / CK-MB
- CBC w dif
- coags
- ABG
- CT spiral
- EKG
- echo?
- # u/s LE

CASE 5: IRREGULAR PERIODS

Doorway Information

Opening Scenario

Kathy Hicks is a 23-year-old woman presents with irregular periods for the past 10 years.

Vital Signs

T 37 C (98.6 F)

BP 120/72 mm Hg   wnl

Pulse 84/min

Respirations 12/min

Examinee Tasks

1. Obtain a focused history.

2. Perform a relevant physical exam. Do not perform rectal, pelvic, genitourinary, female breast, or corneal reflex exam.

3. Discuss your initial diagnostic impression and your workup plan with the patient.

4. After leaving the room, complete your Patient Note.

Communication and Interpersonal Skills Checklist

Fostering the Relationship	Gathering Information	Providing Information
☐ Knocked ☐ Introduced self ☐ Clarified role ☐ Was properly groomed ☐ Made eye contact ☐ Maintained appropriate distance ☐ Displayed confident manner ☐ Showed care and concern ☐ Was respectful and nonjudgmental ☐ Established patient's preferred title ☐ Used proper draping ☐ Focused on patient ☐ Did not interrupt patient ☐ Maintained appropriate and responsive body language	☐ Elicited chief complaint ☐ Established timeline of patient's CC (chief complaint) ☐ Used open-ended question ☐ Used non-leading questions ☐ Used closed-ended questions ☐ Asked one question at a time ☐ Did not use medical jargon ☐ Appropriately used "continuers" ☐ Paraphrased ☐ Appropriately used transitions ☐ Elicited additional concerns ☐ Assessed impact on patient's life ☐ Checked for patient understanding	☐ Summarized significant information ☐ Provided diagnostic impression ☐ Justified diagnosis with evidence from encounter ☐ Assessed patient's need for additional information ☐ Encouraged and answered questions ☐ Assessed patient's comprehension of probable illness

Making Decisions	Supporting Emotions
☐ Clearly stated next steps in management ☐ **Counseled** patient ☐ Agreed to **mutual plan** of action	☐ Actively listened and validated patient's expectations ☐ Showed empathy and used appropriate reassurances ☐ Inquired about patient's support system ☐ Managed the **challenge** (here; patient asked, "Will I have problems getting pregnant?")

History and Physical Examination Checklist

HPI
- ☐ Irregular menstrual periods
- ☐ Duration: 10 years
- ☐ First period at 13
- ☐ Periods were never regular
  - ☐ Every 2-3 mos
- ☐ Gained 15 lbs in last 5 years
  - ☐ Consistent with poor diet
- ☐ No breast tenderness
- ☐ No nipple discharge
- ☐ LMP 8 weeks ago
- ☐ Trying to get pregnant
- ☐ Hirsutism
- ☐ No increased urinary frequency
- ☐ No excessive thirst
- ☐ No cold/heat intolerance
- ☐ No skin or nail changes
- ☐ No constipation

PMH
- ☐ History of menstrual cramps
- ☐ Takes ibuprofen for menstrual cramps
- ☐ Meds: topical benzoyl peroxide for acne, folic acid and multivitamin supplement.
- ☐ Acne since puberty
- ☐ NKDA
- ☐ G0P0
- ☐ No STDs

Family Hx
- ☐ Mother 58 y/o has diabetes
- ☐ Sister 26 y/o had diabetes while pregnant

Social Hx
- ☐ No alcohol
- ☐ No recreational drugs
- ☐ No tobacco use
- ☐ Married
- ☐ Monogamous

Physical Examination

- ☐ Washed hands prior to examination
- ☐ Inspected skin
- ☐ Inspected of abdomen
- ☐ Auscultated 4 quadrants of abdomen
- ☐ Percussed 4 quadrants of abdomen
- ☐ Palpated 4 quadrant of abdomen
  - ☐ Light palpation
  - ☐ Deep palpation if no tenderness upon light palpation
- ☐ Palpated thyroid

(handwritten annotations) abd thyroid; PCOS thyroid dysfunction; pelvic exam serum tests HCG Transabd vag. u/s LH/FSH ratio TSH, T4

Patient Note

History

HPI: 23 y/o woman who has been experiencing irregular menstrual periods for 10 yrs, cycles are every 2-3 mos and menstrual periods have irregular since menarche at age 13. Patient also complains of hirsutism, dysmenorrhea, facial acne and unintentional weight gain of 15 pounds over past 5 years. No breast tenderness, lactation, polydipsia, or change in urinary habits such as frequency has been noted. Pt also denies changes in hair/nails, no cold intolerance

PMH: NKDA, no hospitalizations, surgeries or trauma

Meds: multivitamins with folic acid, ibuprofen taken for dysmenorrhea

FH: father and brother are alive and healthy, mother alive and diabetic, sister with gestational diabetes

OB/Gyn: LMP 8 wks ago; G0 P0

SH: No EtOH/ tobacco/ illicit drugs; diet: processed foods, high in carbohydrate and fat, monogamous with husband, No STDs

---

Physical Examination

T 98.6 F, BP 120/72 mm Hg, pulse 84/min, respirations 12/min

General: alert, conscious and coherent; not in acute distress

HEENT: facial acne noted; neck supple; no thyromegaly

Abd: obese; no abdominal striae; bowel sounds present, tympanic in all 4 quadrants; soft, non-tender, non-distended; no organomegaly

---

Data Interpretation

DIAGNOSIS 1. POLYCYSTIC OVARIAN SYNDROME

History Findings	Physical Exam Findings
Irregular periods for 10 yrs	Facial acne
Hirsutism	No thyromegaly
History of acne	Abd obese
Dysmenorrhea	
Unintentional weight gain of 15 pounds in 5 yrs	
No heat/cold intolerance	
GOPO	
FH of DM	

[handwritten margin notes:]
Exam
- Pelvic vag exam
Labs - TSH, LH, FSH
HbA1c
lipid panel
24hr urinary cortisol
b-HCG
Imaging - transvaginal
u/s

Diagnosis 2. Hypothyroidism

History Findings	Physical Exam Findings
Irregular periods for 10 yrs	Abdominal obesity
Unintentional weight gain of 15 pounds in 5 yrs	

Diagnosis 3. Cushing syndrome

History Findings	Physical Exam Findings
Irregular periods for 10 yrs	Abdominal obesity
Hirsutism	Facial acne
Unintentional weight gain of 15 pounds in 5 yrs	

Diagnostic Studies

Pelvic exam

Serum hCG

Pelvic/transvaginal U/S

OGTT *HbA1c*

Total cholesterol, HDL, LDL, triglycerides *lipidemia*

TSH, LH, FSH

24-hour urinary cortisol excretion

CASE 6: SORE THROAT

Doorway Information

Opening Scenario

Alex Pallon is a 16-year-old male who presents with sore throat for the past 1 day.

Vital Signs

T 38.3 C (101.0 F)

BP 122/60 mm Hg

Pulse 98/min

Respirations 12/min

Oxygen saturation 98% on room air

Examinee Tasks

1. Obtain a focused history.

2. Perform a relevant physical exam. Do not perform rectal, pelvic, genitourinary, female breast, or corneal reflex exam.

3. Discuss your initial diagnostic impression and your workup plan with the patient and his parent.

4. After leaving the room, complete your patient note.

Communication and Interpersonal Skills Checklist

Fostering the Relationship	Gathering Information	Providing Information
☐ Knocked	☐ Elicited chief complaint	☐ Summarized significant information
☐ Introduced self	☐ Established timeline of patient's CC (chief complaint)	☐ Provided diagnostic impression
☐ Clarified role	☐ Used open-ended question	☐ Justified diagnosis with evidence from encounter
☐ Was properly groomed	☐ Used non-leading questions	☐ Assessed patient's need for additional information
☐ Made eye contact	☐ Used closed-ended questions	☐ Encouraged and answered questions
☐ Maintained appropriate distance	☐ Asked one question at a time	☐ Assessed patient's comprehension of probable illness
☐ Displayed confident manner	☐ Did not use medical jargon	
☐ Showed care and concern	☐ Appropriately used "continuers"	
☐ Was respectful and nonjudgmental	☐ Paraphrased	
☐ Established patient's preferred title	☐ Appropriately used transitions	
☐ Used proper draping	☐ Elicited additional concerns	
☐ Focused on patient	☐ Assessed impact on patient's life	
☐ Did not interrupt patient	☐ Checked for patient understanding	
☐ Maintained appropriate and responsive body language		

Making Decisions	Supporting Emotions
☐ Clearly stated next steps in management	☐ Actively listened and validated patient's expectations
☐ **Counseled** patient	☐ Showed empathy and used appropriate reassurances
☐ Agreed to **mutual plan** of action	☐ Inquired about patient's support system
	☐ Managed the **challenge** (here; patient asked, "Can you give me a prescription for antibiotics?")

History and Physical Examination Checklist

HPI
- ☐ Sore throat
- ☐ Sharp pain
  - ☐ Started early this morning
  - ☐ Progressively worse
  - ☐ 8/10 intensity
  - ☐ Greater on the right side
  - ☐ Increased with swallowing
  - ☐ No radiation
- ☐ Symptoms have not improved with rest or ibuprofen
- ☐ Fever (101°F in the morning)
- ☐ Fatigue (left soccer practice early)
- ☐ Chills
- ☐ Headache
- ☐ Nasal discharge
- ☐ No cough
- ☐ No rashes
- ☐ No abdominal pain
- ☐ No nausea or vomiting
- ☐ Sick contacts (soccer teammates)

PMH
- ☐ No similar episodes in the past
- ☐ Meds: no prescription meds or OTC
- ☐ NKDA

Family Hx
- ☐ No relevant family history
- ☐ No siblings

Social Hx
- ☐ No alcohol
- ☐ No recreational drugs
- ☐ Smoked 4 cigarettes over the past 6 mos
- ☐ Not sexually active
- ☐ Physically active (plays soccer)

Physical Examination

- ☐ Washed hands prior to examination
- ☐ Inspected skin for rashes
- ☐ Inspected both nares
- ☐ Inspected, palpated ears bilaterally
- ☐ Performed bilateral otoscopic exam
- ☐ Examined mouth, posterior pharynx and elevation of palate
- ☐ Palpated sinuses for tenderness
- ☐ Palpated posterior auricular lymph nodes
- ☐ Palpated anterior cervical lymph nodes
- ☐ Palpated posterior cervical lymph nodes
- ☐ Palpated submandibular lymph nodes
- ☐ Palpated submental lymph nodes
- ☐ Auscultated both lung fields
- ☐ Percussed thorax

Patient Note

History

HPI: 16 y/o boy c/o sore throat for the past 1 day with 8/10 intensity. He felt tired yesterday and left soccer practice early. A few teammates have also been ill. He states the right throat area hurts more than the left, and the pain is mostly a sharp pain, not radiating anywhere. Pain aggravated by swallowing and alleviated by nothing. He has chills and dull headache but no abdominal pain. No nausea, vomiting or cough. Had fever to 101° F and nasal discharge.

PMH: no previous episodes. NKDA

Meds: none

Hosp/illness/trauma: none

Family Hx: 9 month old brother had a cold recently.

Social History: smoked 4 cigarettes in his whole life. No EtOH or drugs. Lives at home with mother and father. Pt is not sexually active. He plays soccer.

Physical Exam

T 101.0 F, BP 122/60, pulse 98, respirations 12, oxygen saturation 98% on room air

General: patient appears uncomfortable but not in acute distress. AAO x 3

HEENT: Ears (TM visualized, no bulging or erythema, no tenderness elicited). No discharge noted from nares. Throat - erythema noted in posterior pharynx, no exudates noted and tonsils not enlarged. Sinus - no tenderness on palpation. Neck - no LAD

Lungs: CTAB, no wheezes/crepitations/rales/rhonchi

Skin: no erythema or rash noted

Data Interpretation

DIAGNOSIS 1. VIRAL PHARYNGITIS

History Findings	Physical Exam Findings
Sore throat	Erythema on posterior pharynx
Pain aggravated by swallowing	Fever
Fatigue	No lymphadenopathy
Sick contacts	No exudates
Nasal discharge	

DIAGNOSIS 2. STREP PHARYNGITIS

History Findings	Physical Exam Findings
Sore throat	Erythema on posterior pharynx
Pain aggravated by swallowing	Fever
Fatigue	
Sick contacts	
Headache	

DIAGNOSIS 3. INFECTIOUS MONONUCLEOSIS

History Findings	Physical Exam Findings
Sore throat	Erythema on posterior pharynx
Pain aggravated by swallowing	Fever
Fatigue	No nasal discharge
Sick contacts	
Age (primarily young adults)	

Diagnostic Studies

CBC with differential, with peripheral blood smear *mono cells*

Rapid strep test

Throat culture

Monospot test

CASE 7: HEARING LOSS

Doorway Information

Opening Scenario

Ron Ryder is a 43-year-old man who comes to the office today because of hearing loss for the past 5 years.

Vital Signs

T 37 C (98.6 F)

BP 128/72 mm Hg

Pulse 80/min

Respirations 12/min

Examinee Tasks

1. Obtain a focused history.

2. Perform a relevant physical exam. Do not perform rectal, pelvic, genitourinary, or corneal reflex exam.

3. Discuss your initial diagnostic impression and your workup plan with the patient.

4. After leaving the room, complete your Patient Note on the given form.

Communication and Interpersonal Skills Checklist

Fostering the Relationship	Gathering Information	Providing Information
☐ Knocked	☐ Elicited chief complaint	☐ Summarized significant information
☐ Introduced self	☐ Established timeline of patient's CC (chief complaint)	☐ Provided diagnostic impression
☐ Clarified role	☐ Used open-ended question	☐ Justified diagnosis with evidence from encounter
☐ Was properly groomed	☐ Used non-leading questions	☐ Assessed patient's need for additional information
☐ Made eye contact	☐ Used closed-ended questions	☐ Encouraged and answered questions
☐ Maintained appropriate distance	☐ Asked one question at a time	☐ Assessed patient's comprehension of probable illness
☐ Displayed confident manner	☐ Did not use medical jargon	
☐ Showed care and concern	☐ Appropriately used "continuers"	
☐ Was respectful and nonjudgmental	☐ Paraphrased	
☐ Established patient's preferred title	☐ Appropriately used transitions	
☐ Used proper draping	☐ Elicited additional concerns	
☐ Focused on patient	☐ Assessed impact on patient's life	
☐ Did not interrupt patient	☐ Checked for patient understanding	
☐ Maintained appropriate and responsive body language		

Making Decisions	Supporting Emotions
☐ Clearly stated next steps in management	☐ Actively listened and validated patient's expectations
☐ **Counseled** patient	☐ Showed empathy and used appropriate reassurances
☐ Agreed to **mutual plan** of action	☐ Inquired about patient's support system
	☐ Managed the **challenge** (here; patient has difficulty hearing your questions)

History and Physical Examination Checklist

HPI

- ☐ Hearing loss
  - ☐ Bilateral
  - ☐ Noticed 5 years ago
  - ☐ Progressed slowly over the years
  - ☐ Initially a problem with large crowds that have lots of background noise
  - ☐ Lately, can't hear his wife at dinner table
- ☐ No history of ear infections
- ☐ No trauma
- ☐ Uses Q tips to clean wax
  - ☐ No pain
  - ☐ No blood
  - ☐ Minimal wax
- ☐ Tried OTC drops to remove wax
  - ☐ Did not improve hearing
  - ☐ Ears seemed clean of wax
- ☐ Headache
- ☐ No discharge from ear
- ☐ No fever
- ☐ No numbness
- ☐ No tingling
- ☐ No weakness
- ☐ No dizziness
- ☐ No spinning of the room or unsteadiness *vertigo*
- ☐ No ringing in the ears *tinnitus*

PMH

- ☐ No previous hospitalizations or surgeries
- ☐ Meds: no prescription meds
- ☐ Uses aspirin for headaches
- ☐ NKDA

Family Hx

- ☐ No family history of hearing loss

Social Hx

- ☐ He is a farmer
- ☐ Drives loud tractor *exposure*
- ☐ Listens to rock music with head phones
- ☐ Alcohol at social events
- ☐ No recreational drugs
- ☐ No tobacco use
- ☐ Married
- ☐ 3 small children

Physical Examination

SN hearing loss

- ☐ Washed hands prior to examination
- ☐ Tested auditory acuity bilaterally
  - ☐ Cannot hear finger rub bilaterally
- ☐ Inspected external ears
- ☐ Performed otoscopic exam bilaterally
- ☐ Performed Rinne test
  - ☐ Bone conduction is greater than air conduction *SN HL*
- ☐ Performed Weber test
  - ☐ Does not localize to either side
- ☐ Performed posterior auricular, anterior cervical and posterior cervical lymph node exam *CN exam*
- ☐ Observed gait
- ☐ Performed Romberg test

W, Rinne

Patient Note

History

HPI: 43 y/o man presents with bilateral hearing loss for past 5 yrs. Progressively worse; pt initially had trouble hearing in loud social environment but now has trouble hearing his wife at the dinner table. No diurnal variation. Positive headphones use and constant exposure to loud noises. Cleans ears with Q-tips. Has occasional headaches. Denies discharge or blood from the ears. Also denies trauma, fever, pain, numbness/tingling, weakness, tinnitus, vertigo

PMH: no h/o similar cc; no other major illness

Allergies: NKDA

Meds: aspirin PRN for headaches (provides modest relief)

No h/o hospitalizations or surgeries

Family Hx: no similar CC; no other major illness

Social Hx: farmer; 2 beers / wk x 20 yrs; no hx of smoking or recreational drug use. Sexually active with wife only; uses condoms regularly

Physical Examination

T 37 C, BP: 128/72 mm Hg, pulse: 80/min, respirations: 12/min

General: pleasant but cannot hear well despite speaking loudly

HEENT: TM seen; no erythema, polyps or exudates; minimal ear wax; Weber's test not lateralized to any ear; Rinne's test AC > BC, no lymphadenopathy, bilateral hearing loss

CV: normal S1/S2 RRR no M/G/R

Lung: CTABL no wheezes, rhonchi, or rales

Data Interpretation

DIAGNOSIS 1. PRESBYCUSIS

History Findings	Physical Exam Findings
Bilateral hearing loss started 5 yrs ago	Bilateral hearing loss
Progressively worsened	Ear inspection: no erythema, polyps, or exudates; minimal ear wax
Trouble hearing in noisy environment	
Farmer, exposure to loud noises	
Uses headphones	
No fever, pain, numbness/tingling, vertigo	

DIAGNOSIS 2. RUPTURED TYMPANIC MEMBRANE

History Findings	Physical Exam Findings
Hearing loss started 5 yrs ago	Bilateral hearing loss
Farmer, exposure to loud noises	Ear inspection: no erythema, polyps, or exudates; minimal ear wax
Uses headphones	
Cleans ears with Q-tips	
No fever, pain, numbness/tingling, vertigo	
Age	

DIAGNOSIS 3. ASPIRIN TOXICITY

History Findings	Physical Exam Findings
Bilateral hearing loss	Bilateral hearing loss
Hx of aspirin use	Ear inspection: no erythema, polyps, or exudates; minimal ear wax

Diagnostic Studies

CBC w/ differential

Serum salicylate acid level

Audiogram

CASE 8: "SOMETHING IS WRONG WITH MY DAD."

Doorway Information

Opening Scenario

Debby Longo is on the telephone. She is the daughter of Edward Bello, who is 75-years-old. She tells you "something is wrong with my father" after visiting him at his home earlier today.

Vital Signs

Not available

Examinee Tasks

1. Obtain a focused history.

2. You will not be required to perform a physical exam in this case.

3. Discuss your initial diagnostic impression and your workup plan with the patient's daughter.

4. After leaving the room, complete your patient note. Leave the physical exam portion blank.

Communication and Interpersonal Skills Checklist

Fostering the Relationship	Gathering Information	Providing Information
☐ Introduced self ☐ Clarified role ☐ Displayed confident manner ☐ Showed care and concern ☐ Was respectful and nonjudgmental ☐ Established preferred title ☐ Did not interrupt	☐ Elicited chief complaint ☐ Established timeline of patient's CC (chief complaint) ☐ Used open-ended question ☐ Used non-leading questions ☐ Used closed-ended questions ☐ Asked one question at a time ☐ Did not use medical jargon ☐ Appropriately used "continuers" ☐ Paraphrased ☐ Appropriately used transitions ☐ Elicited additional concerns ☐ Assessed impact on patient's life ☐ Checked for understanding	☐ Summarized significant information ☐ Provided diagnostic impression ☐ Justified diagnosis with evidence from encounter ☐ Assessed need for additional information ☐ Encouraged and answered questions ☐ Assessed comprehension of probable illness

Making Decisions	Supporting Emotions
☐ Clearly stated next steps in management ☐ **Counseled** relative ☐ Agreed to **mutual plan** of action	☐ Actively listened and validated expectations ☐ Showed empathy and used appropriate reassurances ☐ Inquired about patient's support system ☐ Managed the **challenge** (here; daughter worried for patient)

STROKE

History and Physical Examination Checklist

HPI
- ☐ Slurred speech
- ☐ Sudden onset
- ☐ Started during breakfast
- ☐ Single episode
- ☐ Duration: 20 mins
- ☐ Difficulty opening a jar of jelly
- ☐ Unable to hold a cup of coffee
- ☐ Patient stumbled when he tried to stand
- ☐ Difficulty moving right leg
- ☐ + headache
- ☐ No dysphagia
- ☐ No loss of consciousness
- ☐ No bowel or bladder incontinence
- ☐ No visual problems
- ☐ No loss of sensation
- ☐ No jerky movements of limbs
- ☐ No fever
- ☐ No confusion
- ☐ Drooping face

PMH
- ☐ High cholesterol
- ☐ Last test 6 mos ago 110 mg/dl LDL
- ☐ No HTN
- ☐ No diabetes
- ☐ No heart disease
- ☐ No history of stroke
- ☐ No previous surgery or hospitalization
- ☐ NKDA
- ☐ Meds: aspirin and atorvastatin

Family Hx
- ☐ Father died of stroke at age 92
- ☐ Social Hx
- ☐ Retired malpractice lawyer
- ☐ No smoking
- ☐ Alcohol 1-2 times per month
- ☐ Plays golf on weekends

Physical Examination

No physical exam

Patient Note

History

HPI: Hx provided by daughter on phone. 75 y/o man c/o slurred speech for 20 min. Sudden onset yesterday morning. No clear precipitating factor. Had trouble picking up jar of jelly with R hand. He stumbled getting out of chair due to difficulty moving his R leg but did not fall. His symptoms resolved spontaneously. He also reported a headache. No difficulty swallowing. His wife noticed his face looked "little different" during the episode. No further episodes. Negative h/o of fever, confusion, vision changes, loss of sensation, no bowel or bladder incontinence, no tonic-clonic movements.

PMH: h/o hyperlipidemia; no h/o similar episodes in past; last physical 6 mos ago–lipid panel normal.

Meds: Aspirin daily, atorvastatin compliant; NKDA ; no h/o hosp or surgeries; sleep not disturbed

Family Hx: no similar CC; no other major illness

Social Hx: he drinks 1-2 drinks/month; no h/o smoking or rec drugs

Physical Exam

None

Data Interpretation

DIAGNOSIS 1. TRANSIENT ISCHEMIC ATTACK

History Findings	Physical Exam Findings
Sudden onset of slurring speech	
Duration 20 min	
R hand weakness	
Transient R leg weakness	
Face looked "little different"	
No h/o fever, confusion, LOC, incontinence, tonic-clonic movements	

DIAGNOSIS 2. CEREBROVASCULAR ACCIDENT

History Findings	Physical Exam Findings
Sudden onset of slurred speech	
R hand weakness	
Transient R leg weakness	
Face looked "little different"	
Negative h/o fever, tonic-clonic movements	
Elevated cholesterol	

Diagnostic Studies

Physical examination

Cholesterol, HDL, LDL, triglycerides, CBC, electrolytes, glucose, PT, PTT

EKG

Carotid U/S

CT scan of head without contrast

Echocardiogram

MRI/MRA of brain

CASE 9: SEVERE HEADACHE

Doorway Information

Opening Scenario

Patrick Davis is a 45-year-old man who comes to the ER because of a severe headache for the past 4 hours.

Vital Signs

T 37.8 C (100 F)

BP 169/108 mm Hg

Pulse 48/min

Respirations 12/min

[handwritten: HTN brady — Cushing's reflex]

Examinee Tasks

1. Obtain a focused history.

2. Perform a relevant physical exam. Do not perform rectal, pelvic, genitourinary, or corneal reflex exam.

3. Discuss your initial diagnostic impression and your workup plan with the patient.

4. After leaving the room, complete the patient note.

Communication and Interpersonal Skills Checklist		
Fostering the Relationship	**Gathering Information**	**Providing Information**
☐ Knocked ☐ Introduced self ☐ Clarified role ☐ Was properly groomed ☐ Made eye contact ☐ Maintained appropriate distance ☐ Displayed confident manner ☐ Showed care and concern ☐ Was respectful and nonjudgmental ☐ Established patient's preferred title ☐ Used proper draping ☐ Focused on patient ☐ Did not interrupt patient ☐ Maintained appropriate and responsive body language	☐ Elicited chief complaint ☐ Established timeline of patient's CC (chief complaint) ☐ Used open-ended question ☐ Used non-leading questions ☐ Used closed-ended questions ☐ Asked one question at a time ☐ Did not use medical jargon ☐ Appropriately used "continuers" ☐ Paraphrased ☐ Appropriately used transitions ☐ Elicited additional concerns ☐ Assessed impact on patient's life ☐ Checked for patient understanding	☐ Summarized significant information ☐ Provided diagnostic impression ☐ Justified diagnosis with evidence from encounter ☐ Assessed patient's need for additional information ☐ Encouraged and answered questions ☐ Assessed patient's comprehension of probable illness
Making Decisions	**Supporting Emotions**	
☐ Clearly stated next steps in management ☐ **Counseled** patient ☐ Agreed to **mutual plan** of action	☐ Actively listened and validated patient's expectations ☐ Showed empathy and used appropriate reassurances ☐ Inquired about patient's support system ☐ Managed the **challenge** (here; patient asked, "Can you make it stop?")	

History and Physical Examination Checklist

HPI

- ☐ Headache
  - ☐ 10/10 intensity
  - ☐ Persistent
  - ☐ Radiation to neck and back
  - ☐ Started while coaching his daughter's Little League game
- ☐ Duration: 4 hours
- ☐ Worse with cough
- ☐ Worse with movement of head
- ☐ Nausea
- ☐ No vomiting
- ☐ No LOC
- ☐ No Trauma
- ☐ No seizures
- ☐ No fever
- ☐ No chills
- ☐ No photophobia
- ☐ No confusion
- ☐ No changes in vision
- ☐ No recent illness
- ☐ No sick contacts

PMH

- ☐ No similar episodes in the past
- ☐ No hospitalizations or surgeries
- ☐ Meds: 400mg of ibuprofen earlier
- ☐ NKDA

Family Hx

- ☐ No family history of stroke, vascular disease or heart disease
- ☐ Maternal uncle has polycystic kidney disease on hemodialysis

Social Hx

- ☐ Alcohol 1-2 glasses/5 days a week
- ☐ Snorts cocaine on most weekends
- ☐ No IV drug use
- ☐ Smokes
  - ☐ 1-2 pack/day
  - ☐ 10 years
- ☐ Married, sexually active with wife only
- ☐ Works as a bartender at a local bar

Physical Examination

- ☐ Washed hands prior to examination
- ☐ Performed Mental status exam
- ☐ Performed inspection of head
- ☐ Performed palpation of head
- ☐ Performed fundoscopic exam
- ☐ Examined CNII–XII
- ☐ Assessed motor strength bilaterally
- ☐ Examined DTRs
- ☐ Checked sensation with at least 2 modalities (light, sharp/dull, proprioception)
- ☐ Assessed cerebellar function (dysmetria, dysdiadochokinesia or Romberg)
- ☐ Examined for Babinski reflex
- ☐ Performed Brudzinski or Kernig test

Patient Note

History

HPI: 45 y/o man who presents with a severe headache for the past 4 hours. He reports having a generalized headache. The headache is sharp with intensity of 10/10, radiates down his neck and spine, is aggravated by movement and he has no relief with OTC analgesics and is assoc with nausea. He describes it as the "worst headache of my life." He denies vomiting, fevers, chills, sick contact, seizures, confusion, recent URI, vertigo, trauma, tinnitus or loss of consciousness. He admits to using cocaine on most weekends, but denies other drug use. He has a family history of polycystic kidney disease.

PMH/PSHx: No h/o similar symptoms in the past, no other major illness, No h/o hospitalizations or surgeries.

Allergies: NKDA

Meds: Ibuprofen OTC for relief; no regular meds or supplements

Family Hx: No similar CC; uncle on dialysis for PCKD

Social Hx: 1 beer everyday x 10 yrs; 1-2 packs of cigs/day x 10 yrs; h/o cocaine snorting - no IVDU, sexually active with wife only; uses condoms regularly

Physical Examination

BP 169/108 mm Hg, pulse 48/min, T 37.8 C, respirations 12/min

Appears confused and in moderate distress

A&O x 2: can't remember date

Eyes: visual acuity, visual fields and EOM are intact; no papilledema or optic disc blurring on fundoscopy

CN II–XII intact

LE: motor: 5/5 b/I DTR: 2+ throughout

Sensory: light, sharp/dull & proprioception intact b/I

No dysmetria, dysdiadochokinesia

Babinski negative, Brudzinski +

Data Interpretation

DIAGNOSIS 1. RUPTURED CEREBRAL ANEURYSM

History Findings	Physical Exam Findings
Generalized headache	Hypertensive, afebrile
Sharp with intensity of 10/10 "worst headache of life"	A&O x 2: can't remember date
Aggravated by movement and no relief with analgesics	Brudzinski test: positive
Associated with nausea	
Pain radiating down neck and spine	
No hx of fevers, chills, sick contact, trauma	
Family h/o PCKD	
1–2 packs of cig/day	

DIAGNOSIS 2. COCAINE-INDUCED HYPERTENSIVE INTRACRANIAL HEMORRHAGE

History Findings	Physical Exam Findings
Generalized headache	Hypertensive
Sharp with intensity of 10/10 "worst headache of life"	A&O x 2 : can't remember date
Aggravated by movement and no relief with OTC pain meds	Brudzinski test: positive
Assoc with nausea	
Negative h/o fevers, chills, sick contact, recent URI, trauma	
h/o cocaine-snorting	

DIAGNOSIS 3. MENINGITIS

History Findings	Physical Exam Findings
Generalized headache	Hypertensive, bradycardia
Severe headache	A&O x 2 : can't remember date
Aggravated by movement and no relief with OTC pain meds	No papilledema or optic disc blurring on fundoscopy
Assoc with nausea	Brudzinski test: positive

Diagnostic Studies

CBC w diff

Urine toxicology

CT head without contrast

Lumbar puncture

MRI brain, MRA brain

- CBC
- utox
- CT head → MRI
- LP w/ CSF analysis

CASE 10: SEVERE ABDOMINAL PAIN

Doorway Information

Opening Scenario

Michelle Thompson is a 31-year-old woman who comes to the ER because of severe abdominal pain for the past 5 hours.

Vital Signs

T 38.3 C (101.0 F)

BP 102/60 mm Hg

Pulse 109/min

Respirations 27/min

Examinee Tasks

1. Obtain a focused history.

2. Perform a relevant physical exam. Do not perform rectal, pelvic, genitourinary, female breast, or corneal reflex exam.

3. Discuss your initial diagnostic impression and your workup plan with the patient.

4. After leaving the room, complete your patient note.

Communication and Interpersonal Skills Checklist

Fostering the Relationship	Gathering Information	Providing Information
☐ Knocked	☐ Elicited chief complaint	☐ Summarized significant information
☐ Introduced self	☐ Established timeline of patient's CC (chief complaint)	☐ Provided diagnostic impression
☐ Clarified role	☐ Used open-ended question	☐ Justified diagnosis with evidence from encounter
☐ Was properly groomed	☐ Used non-leading questions	☐ Assessed patient's need for additional information
☐ Made eye contact	☐ Used closed-ended questions	☐ Encouraged and answered questions
☐ Maintained appropriate distance	☐ Asked one question at a time	☐ Assessed patient's comprehension of probable illness
☐ Displayed confident manner	☐ Did not use medical jargon	
☐ Showed care and concern	☐ Appropriately used "continuers"	
☐ Was respectful and nonjudgmental	☐ Paraphrased	
☐ Established patient's preferred title	☐ Appropriately used transitions	
☐ Used proper draping	☐ Elicited additional concerns	
☐ Focused on patient	☐ Assessed impact on patient's life	
☐ Did not interrupt patient	☐ Checked for patient understanding	
☐ Maintained appropriate and responsive body language		

Making Decisions	Supporting Emotions
☐ Clearly stated next steps in management	☐ Actively listened and validated patient's expectations
☐ **Counseled** patient	☐ Showed empathy and used appropriate reassurances
☐ Agreed to **mutual plan** of action	☐ Inquired about patient's support system
	☐ Managed the **challenge** (here; patient asked, "Will I need surgery?")

History and Physical Examination Checklist

HPI

- ☐ Abdominal pain
  - ☐ LUQ and RUQ
  - ☐ Dull
  - ☐ 10/10 intensity
  - ☐ Constant
  - ☐ Radiates to the back
- ☐ Duration: 5 hours
- ☐ Aspirin did not alleviate her symptoms
- ☐ Leaning forward alleviates pain
- ☐ Laying supine exacerbates pain
- ☐ No fever
- ☐ No chills
- ☐ No diarrhea
- ☐ No cough
- ☐ No chest pain
- ☐ No dark stools
- ☐ No sick contacts
- ☐ 3 episodes of emesis today
  - ☐ Non-bloody
  - ☐ Non-bilious

PMH

- ☐ 1 similar episode in the past
  - ☐ 2 years ago
  - ☐ Admitted to the intensive care unit
  - ☐ Does not recall her diagnosis or treatment
- ☐ Recurrent urinary tract infections
- ☐ No surgeries
- ☐ Meds: no prescription meds
- ☐ NKDA
- ☐ No children
- ☐ LMP 10 days ago

Family Hx

- ☐ Mother with hx of type 2 diabetes
- ☐ Father with hx of high BP
- ☐ Both mother and maternal aunt with hx of gallstone disease

Social Hx

- ☐ Heavy alcohol use
- ☐ 5-6 drinks daily on weekends
- ☐ Last alcoholic beverage 5 days ago
- ☐ No recreational drugs
- ☐ Does not smoke
- ☐ Sexually active with boyfriend only
- ☐ Uses condoms
- ☐ No history of STDs

Physical Examination

- ☐ Washed hands prior to examination
- ☐ Inspected of abdomen
- ☐ Auscultated 4 quadrants +epigastric
- ☐ Percussed 4 quadrants + epigastric
- ☐ Palpated 4 quadrants
  - ☐ + voluntary guarding
  - ☐ No rebound tenderness
- ☐ Assessed liver and spleen span
- ☐ Inspected skin
- ☐ Inspected sclera
- ☐ Assessed rebound tenderness
- ☐ Tested for Murphy's sign
  - ☐ Murphy sign is absent
  - ☐ Rovsing, obturator, and iliopsoas signs also negative

Patient Note

History

HPI: 31 y/o woman c/o severe abdominal pain for 5 hrs. Sudden onset. 10/10 severity. constant and dull. LUQ and RUQ, radiating to the back. Aspirin did not relieve symptoms. Leaning forward helps alleviate the pain and laying supine exacerbates it. She had 3 episodes of non-bloody, non-bilious emesis. No fever, chills, diarrhea, cough, chest pain, or dark stools. No recent sick contacts.

PMH: similar symptoms 2 yrs ago, admitted to ICU, h/o frequent UTIs, NKDA. No new medications and no herbal medications.

FHx: mother has type 2 diabetes, gallstone disease; father has HTN, maternal aunt w/ gallstone disease

SHx: sexually active, monogamous, regular condom use, no STDs, pt drinks 5-6 drinks daily on weekends, no recreational drug use, no tobacco use.

Physical Exam

T 101.0 F; BP102/60 mm Hg; pulse 109/min; respirations 27/min

GA: alert, conscious and coherent; anxious and uncomfortable; in moderate distress

HEENT: no scleral icterus,

Abdominal: no scars or bruises; tympanic in all 4 quadrants and epigastric area; diffusely tender in epigastrium, RUQ, and LUQ, voluntary guarding; no rebound tenderness; no hepatosplenomegaly, bowel sounds present. Negative Murphy, psoas, obturator, and Rovsing signs

Skin: no jaundice

Data Interpretation

DIAGNOSIS 1: ACUTE PANCREATITIS, DUE TO ALCOHOL OR GALLSTONE

History Findings	Physical Exam Findings
Sudden onset of upper abdominal pain	Tachycardia
Constant, dull	Fever
Radiation to back, alleviated by leaning forward	Tachypnea
Family h/o gallstone disease	Voluntary guarding
Heavy alcohol use	Tenderness in epigastrium and RUQ
Three episodes of vomiting	

DIAGNOSIS 2: CHOLECYSTITIS

History Findings	Physical Exam Findings
Sudden onset of upper abdominal pain	Tachycardic 109/min
Constant	Fever
Family h/o gallstone disease	RUQ and epigastric tenderness
Three episodes of vomiting	Voluntary guarding

DIAGNOSIS 3: PEPTIC ULCER DISEASE

History Findings	Physical Exam Findings
Sudden onset of constant upper abdominal pain	Tachycardia
Heavy alcohol use	Diffusely tender, especially in epigastrium and RUQ
NSAID use	Guarding

Diagnostic Studies

Rectal exam: fecal occult blood

Serum electrolytes, CBC with diff

Amylase

Lipase

AST, ALT, glucose, calcium

Abdominal ultrasound

Esophagogastroduodenoscopy

labs
- CBC w/ dif
- BMP
- Ca
- lipase, amylase
- ALP AST ALT + bili
GGT
- ETOH levels
- utox
- FOBT
+ imaging
CT abd
RUQ u/s
EGD if other w/u⊖

CASE 11: CHRONIC DIARRHEA

Doorway Information

Opening Scenario

Bernice Roth is a 30-year-old woman who presents with complaints of recurrent diarrheal episodes for the past year.

Vital Signs

T 37.9 C (100.2 F)

BP 128/92 mm Hg

Pulse 80/min

Respirations 16/min

Examinee Tasks

1. Obtain a focused history.

2. Perform a relevant physical exam. Do not perform rectal, pelvic, genitourinary, or corneal reflex exam.

3. Discuss your initial diagnostic impression and your workup plan with the patient.

IBD
celiacs
IBS

Communication and Interpersonal Skills Checklist

Fostering the Relationship	Gathering Information	Providing Information
☐ Knocked	☐ Elicited chief complaint	☐ Summarized significant information
☐ Introduced self	☐ Established timeline of patient's CC (chief complaint)	☐ Provided diagnostic impression
☐ Clarified role	☐ Used open-ended question	☐ Justified diagnosis with evidence from encounter
☐ Was properly groomed	☐ Used non-leading questions	☐ Assessed patient's need for additional information
☐ Made eye contact	☐ Used closed-ended questions	☐ Encouraged and answered questions
☐ Maintained appropriate distance	☐ Asked one question at a time	☐ Assessed patient's comprehension of probable illness
☐ Displayed confident manner	☐ Did not use medical jargon	
☐ Showed care and concern	☐ Appropriately used "continuers"	
☐ Was respectful and nonjudgmental	☐ Paraphrased	
☐ Established patient's preferred title	☐ Appropriately used transitions	
☐ Used proper draping	☐ Elicited additional concerns	
☐ Focused on patient	☐ Assessed impact on patient's life	
☐ Did not interrupt patient	☐ Checked for patient understanding	
☐ Maintained appropriate and responsive body language		

Making Decisions	Supporting Emotions
☐ Clearly stated next steps in management	☐ Actively listened and validated patient's expectations
☐ **Counseled** patient	☐ Showed empathy and used appropriate reassurances
☐ Agreed to **mutual plan** of action	☐ Inquired about patient's support system
	☐ Managed the **challenge** (here, patient asked, "Can you help?")

History and Physical Examination Checklist

HPI

- ☐ Recurrent episodes of diarrhea
- ☐ Duration: 1 year
- ☐ Waxes and wanes
- ☐ 10-20 bowel movements per day when most frequent
- ☐ Fecal incontinence (finds stool in underwear)
- ☐ Blood
  - ☐ Occasionally
  - ☐ Mixed with stool
- ☐ Large amounts of mucus
- ☐ Abdominal pain
  - ☐ 4/10 intensity
  - ☐ Crampy
- ☐ Intermittent fevers
- ☐ 20 lb weight loss
- ☐ Intermittent joint pain
  - ☐ Knees
- ☐ No visual changes
- ☐ No red eyes
- ☐ No skin rashes
- ☐ No known sick contacts
- ☐ No post prandial bloating
- ☐ No oral ulcers
- ☐ Recent travel to Israel

PMH

- ☐ Perianal fistula
  - ☐ Repaired 1.5 years ago
- ☐ Meds: no prescription meds
- ☐ NKDA

Family Hx

- ☐ Uncle had "problem with his intestines" which required surgery and resection

Social Hx

- ☐ Full time rabbinical student
- ☐ Sexually active and monogamous with husband
- ☐ Has 2 healthy children
- ☐ No drugs
- ☐ No smoking
- ☐ No alcohol use

Physical Examination

- ☐ Washed hands prior to examination
- ☐ Inspected abdomen
- ☐ Auscultated abdomen in 4 quadrants
- ☐ Percussed abdomen in all 4 quadrants
- ☐ Lightly palpated abdomen in all 4 quadrants
- ☐ Deeply palpated abdomen in all 4quadrants
  - ☐ Mildly tender to palpation in the RLQ
  - ☐ No rebound tenderness
  - ☐ No guarding
- ☐ Assessed abdomen for rebound tenderness and guarding
- ☐ Inspected eyes for evidence of uveitis
- ☐ Examined oral mucosa
- ☐ Inspected skin for any lesions
- ☐ Examined joints for evidence of inflammation

Patient Note

History

HPI: 30 y/o woman presents with recurrent episodes of diarrhea for the past 1 year. The diarrhea occasionally contains gross blood and mucus. She can have as many as 10-20 BMs daily with some fecal incontinence. She reports associated abdominal pain which is crampy, located in lower abd without radiation. She also has associated joint pains. ROS also notable for occasional fevers and 20 lb weight loss. She denies rash, visual changes, red eye.

PMH: h/o perianal fistula

Allergies: no known drug allergies

Medications: no Rx, OTC medications, or supplements

FH: Uncle had GI illness with "partial gut resection." No h/o colon cancer in family

SH: no EtOH/cig/drug use

Married, has 2 healthy children. Rabbinic student

Physical Examination

VS: T 100.2 F, BP 128/92 mm Hg, pulse 80/min, respirations 16/min

GA: thin and pale, NAD

Abd: BS (+) x 4Q; tympanic x 4Q;: mild tenderness to palpation RLQ, no guarding or rebound tenderness, no palpable masses, non-distended

Ext: no cyanosis, clubbing, edema; no effusion/inflammation in joints

Eyes: Sclera anicteric, PEERLA, EOMI

Oropharynx: moist mucous membranes, no oral ulcers

Data Interpretation

DIAGNOSIS 1. CROHN'S DISEASE

History Findings	Physical Exam Findings
Diarrhea x 1 yr; 10 20 BMs/day	Fever
Abdominal cramping	Mild tenderness to palpation RLQ
h/o fecal incontinence	
h/o perianal fistula	
20-lb weight loss	
Fever	
Arthralgias	
Uncle had GI illness w/ "partial gut resection"	

DIAGNOSIS 2. ULCERATIVE COLITIS

History Findings	Physical Exam Findings
Diarrhea x 1 year, 10–20 BMs/day	Fever
h/o fecal incontinence	Mild tenderness to palpation RLQ
20-lb weight loss	
Occasional gross blood	
Fever	
Arthralgias	
Uncle had GI illness with "partial gut resection"	

DIAGNOSIS 3. CHRONIC INFECTIOUS DIARRHEA (AMEBIASIS, YERSINIOSIS)

History Findings	Physical Exam Findings
Diarrhea x 1 year, 10–20 BMs/day	Fever
Occasional gross blood	Mild tenderness to palpation RLQ
h/o fecal incontinence	
Fever	

Diagnostic Studies

Rectal exam

CBC w/differential

ESR, serum albumin

ASCA, pANCA

Colonoscopy   WBC

Stool culture, ova and parasites, fecal leukocytes, stool antigen for *E. histolytica*

CASE 12: ABDOMINAL PAIN AND YELLOW SKIN

Doorway Information

Opening Scenario

Jerry Matthews is a 55-year-old man who presents because of worsening abdominal pain and yellow skin for the past 2 weeks.

Vital Signs

T 37.1 C (98.8 F)

BP 118/72 mm Hg

Pulse 95/min

Respirations 14/min

Examinee Tasks

1. Obtain a focused history.

2. Perform a relevant physical exam. Do not perform rectal, pelvic, genitourinary, or corneal reflex exam.

3. Discuss your initial diagnostic impression and your workup plan with the patient.

4. After leaving the room, complete your patient note on the given form.

Communication and Interpersonal Skills Checklist		
Fostering the Relationship	**Gathering Information**	**Providing Information**
☐ Knocked ☐ Introduced self ☐ Clarified role ☐ Was properly groomed ☐ Made eye contact ☐ Maintained appropriate distance ☐ Displayed confident manner ☐ Showed care and concern ☐ Was respectful and nonjudgmental ☐ Established patient's preferred title ☐ Used proper draping ☐ Focused on patient ☐ Did not interrupt patient ☐ Maintained appropriate and responsive body language	☐ Elicited chief complaint ☐ Established timeline of patient's CC (chief complaint) ☐ Used open-ended question ☐ Used non-leading questions ☐ Used closed-ended questions ☐ Asked one question at a time ☐ Did not use medical jargon ☐ Appropriately used "continuers" ☐ Paraphrased ☐ Appropriately used transitions ☐ Elicited additional concerns ☐ Assessed impact on patient's life ☐ Checked for patient understanding	☐ Summarized significant information ☐ Provided diagnostic impression ☐ Justified diagnosis with evidence from encounter ☐ Assessed patient's need for additional information ☐ Encouraged and answered questions ☐ Assessed patient's comprehension of probable illness
Making Decisions	**Supporting Emotions**	
☐ Clearly stated next steps in management ☐ **Counseled** patient ☐ Agreed to **mutual plan** of action	☐ Actively listened and validated patient's expectations ☐ Showed empathy and used appropriate reassurances ☐ Inquired about patient's support system ☐ Managed the **challenge** (here; patient asked, "This is because of my drinking, isn't it?")	

History and Physical Examination Checklist	
HPI	**PMH**
☐ Abdominal pain	☐ History of degenerative joint disease
☐ Duration: 2 weeks	☐ Knees
☐ Progressively worsening	☐ Takes large amounts of acetaminophen for the pain
☐ RUQ	☐ Meds: no prescription meds
☐ Dull	☐ NKDA
☐ 5/10 intensity	**Family Hx**
☐ Constant	☐ No significant family history
☐ No radiation	☐ Except an uncle who died of liver problems
☐ Jaundice	☐ Not been around anyone sick recently
☐ Dark urine	**Social Hx**
☐ Light colored stools	☐ Currently unemployed
☐ Fatigue	☐ Lives in homeless shelter
☐ no nausea	☐ Denies smoking
☐ No vomiting	☐ Alcohol use
☐ No diarrhea	☐ Heavy drinker
☐ No fever	☐ Past 5-10 years
☐ No bruising	☐ Just finished a week-long binge
☐ No rectal bleeding or hematemesis	☐ Denies current drug use
☐ No history of confusion	☐ Used to inject heroin
☐ No history of distended abdomen	☐ Not current sexually active
☐ 20 lb weight loss	☐ Numerous past sexual partners
☐ Over the last 2 mos	☐ Does not use condoms regularly
☐ Doesn't feel hungry	☐ Unsure of HIV status
☐ Drinks instead	☐ No recent travel

Physical Examination	
☐ Washed hands prior to examination	☐ Deeply palpated abdomen in all non-tender quadrants
☐ Checked for scleral icterus (+)	☐ Tenderness in RUQ
☐ Inspected abdomen	☐ Checked for splenomegaly
☐ Non-distended	☐ Spleen is not palpable
☐ Inspected skin for signs/stigmata of liver disease	☐ Checked for presence of Murphy sign (−)
☐ Auscultated abdomen in all 4 quadrants	☐ Checked for rebound tenderness
☐ Percussed abdomen in all 4 quadrants	☐ Examined for ascites
☐ Measured liver span	☐ No shifting dullness or fluid wave
☐ Liver edge is palpable 6-7 cm below costal margin	☐ Checked extremities for edema
☐ Lightly palpated abdomen in all 4 quadrants	☐ Checked palms for erythema
	☐ Checked skin for spider angiomata

Patient Note

History

HPI: 55 y/o man presents with worsening abdominal pain and yellow skin for 2 weeks. The pain is located in the RUQ, is 5/10, dull, constant, and non-radiating. Associated symptoms include tea-colored urine and light colored stool. He also notes a 2 month history of 20lb weight loss, anorexia and fatigue. He has no nausea, vomiting, diarrhea or fevers. He is a heavy alcohol drinker and recently binge drank. He also reports a history of degenerative joint disease of the knees and has been taking acetaminophen on a daily basis.

PMH: no prior occurrences of similar event, knee osteoarthritis, h/o alcoholism x 5–10 yrs

Allergies: NKDA

Medications: Acetaminophen

FH: Uncle: liver failure

SH: Homeless, lives in shelter, unemployed. Non-smoker. Heavy alcohol use, last drink today after week long binge. Past h/o IVDU (heroin). Not currently sexually active. No past h/o STDs, multiple sexual partners without condoms

Physical Examination

VS: T 37.1 C, BP 118/72 mm Hg, pulse 95/min, respirations 14/min

Gen: malnourished, appears older than stated age, NAD

HEENT: scleral icterus, dry mucous membranes

Abd: BS (+) x 4, tympanic to percussion x 4Q, marked hepatomegaly. No splenomegaly. RUQ tenderness. No guarding, rebound, or Murphy's sign. No shifting dullness or fluid wave

Skin: no lesions or spider angiomata

Ext: no palmar erythema, no edema

Data Interpretation

Diagnosis 1. Alcoholic hepatitis

History Findings	Physical Exam Findings
Jaundice	Malnourished, NAD
RUQ pain	Jaundice, scleral icterus
Tea-colored urine, light colored stool	RUQ tenderness
h/o alcoholism	No Murphy's sign
Homeless, lives in shelter, unemployed	Tender hepatomegaly
Fatigue	

DIAGNOSIS 2. VIRAL HEPATITIS (A, B OR C))

History Findings	Physical Exam Findings
Jaundice	Malnourished, NAD
Weight loss, malaise, anorexia	Jaundice, scleral icterus
Tea-colored urine, light colored stool	No Murphy's sign
Homeless, lives in shelter	
Past h/o IVDU (heroin)	
Multiple sexual partners without condoms	

DIAGNOSIS 3. ACETAMINOPHEN TOXICITY

History Findings	Physical Exam Findings
Jaundice	NAD
Tea-colored urine, light colored stool	Jaundice, scleral icterus
RUQ pain	RUQ tenderness
Medications: acetaminophen	No Murphy's sign
Decreased appetite	Hepatomegaly

Diagnostic Studies

CBC w/ differential

AST, ALT, alkaline phosphatase, total bilirubin, direct bilirubin, indirect bilirubin, albumin, total protein

PT/INR, PTT

HAV IgM, HCV antibody, HCV PCR, HBsAg, HBsAb, HBV core Ab IgM

Acetaminophen level

RUQ U/S

CASE 13: COUGH AND FEVER

Opening Scenario

Paul Lambert is a 66-year-old man who presents to the ER complaining of cough and fever.

Vital Signs

T 38.3 C (101.0 F)

BP 146/90 mm Hg

Pulse 107/min

Respirations 28/min

SpO2 90% on room air

Examinee Tasks

1. Obtain a focused history.

2. Perform a relevant physical exam. Do not perform rectal, pelvic, genitourinary, or corneal reflex exam.

3. Discuss your initial diagnostic impression and your workup plan with the patient.

4. After leaving the room, complete your Patient Note on the given form.

Communication and Interpersonal Skills Checklist

Fostering the Relationship	Gathering Information	Providing Information
☐ Knocked ☐ Introduced self ☐ Clarified role ☐ Was properly groomed ☐ Made eye contact ☐ Maintained appropriate distance ☐ Displayed confident manner ☐ Showed care and concern ☐ Was respectful and nonjudgmental ☐ Established patient's preferred title ☐ Used proper draping ☐ Focused on patient ☐ Did not interrupt patient ☐ Maintained appropriate and responsive body language	☐ Elicited chief complaint ☐ Established timeline of patient's CC (chief complaint) ☐ Used open-ended question ☐ Used non-leading questions ☐ Used closed-ended questions ☐ Asked one question at a time ☐ Did not use medical jargon ☐ Appropriately used "continuers" ☐ Paraphrased ☐ Appropriately used transitions ☐ Elicited additional concerns ☐ Assessed impact on patient's life ☐ Checked for patient understanding	☐ Summarized significant information ☐ Provided diagnostic impression ☐ Justified diagnosis with evidence from encounter ☐ Assessed patient's need for additional information ☐ Encouraged and answered questions ☐ Assessed patient's comprehension of probable illness

Making Decisions	Supporting Emotions
☐ Clearly stated next steps in management ☐ **Counseled** patient ☐ Agreed to **mutual plan** of action	☐ Actively listened and validated patient's expectations ☐ Showed empathy and used appropriate reassurances ☐ Inquired about patient's support system ☐ Managed the **challenge** (here; patient asked, "is it serious?")

History and Physical Examination Checklist	

HPI
- ☐ Chronic cough
  - ☐ Duration: 6 mos
  - ☐ Productive
    - ☐ 1 teaspoonful
- ☐ Blood streaks on sputum
- ☐ Cough worse over past 3 days
  - ☐ Currently a greenish-yellow sputum
- ☐ Shortness of breath
  - ☐ When climbing up stairs
- ☐ Fever
  - ☐ Low grade
- ☐ No chills
- ☐ No night sweats
- ☐ Wheezing
  - ☐ Intermittent
  - ☐ Requires albuterol inhaler
- ☐ No chest pain
- ☐ No sick contacts
- ☐ No travel
- ☐ No halitosis
- ☐ Fatigue
- ☐ Usual exercise tolerance lower
- ☐ Weight loss
  - ☐ 20 lbs
  - ☐ Over 3 mos

PMH
- ☐ COPD
- ☐ 2 previous episodes of pneumonia
  - ☐ Treated
  - ☐ 1 required hospitalization
- ☐ Hypertension
- ☐ No surgery
- ☐ Meds
  - ☐ Atenolol
  - ☐ Ipratropium inhaler daily
  - ☐ Albuterol (as needed)
- ☐ NKDA

Family Hx
- ☐ No significant family history
- ☐ Not been around anyone sick recently

Social Hx
- ☐ 40 pack year hx of smoking tobacco
  - ☐ Stopped smoking 3 days ago (due to illness)
- ☐ No alcohol use
- ☐ No drug use
- ☐ Retired postal worker

Physical Examination
- ☐ Washed hands prior to examination
- ☐ Assessed the patient for respiratory distress
- ☐ Performed a lymph node exam of the neck
- ☐ Assessed neck for JVD
- ☐ Performed inspection of chest
  - ☐ Chest wall appears symmetrical
- ☐ Performed percussion of lungs
- ☐ Assessed for egophony and tactile fremitus
  - ☐ decreased tactile fremitus
- ☐ Auscultated lungs
  - ☐ Coughs when asked to breathe deeply
  - ☐ Scattered expiratory wheezes bilaterally, but no crackles or rales
- ☐ Examined extremities for cyanosis/clubbing/edema
- ☐ Examined oropharynx
- ☐ Performed cardiac auscultation
- ☐ Assessed PMI

Patient Note

History

HPI: 66 y/o woman with past medical history notable for COPD with chronic bronchitis characterized by productive cough, presents to the ER with worsening cough and fevers x3 days. The cough is now productive of increasing amounts of greenish-yellow sputum, sometimes blood-tinged. He has low grade fevers but no shaking chills. He has associated intermittent chest tightness and wheezing with increased use of his albuterol inhaler and increased DOE. Other notable ROS include chronic fatigue and weight loss of 20 lbs over the last 3 mos. He has a 40 pack year smoking history. He denies sick contacts, travel, or chest pain.

PMH: h/o pneumonia x 2, COPD, HTN, no surgeries

Allergies: NKDA

Meds: Atenolol, , ipratropium, albuterol prn

FHx: no major illness

S Hx: 1 pack/day x 40 yrs; no h/o EtoH or rec drugs

Physical Exam

BP 146/90 mm Hg, pulse 107/min, T 38.3 C, respirations 28/min, SpO2: 90% on room air

Gen: appears anxious, uncomfortable and in mild respiratory distress

OP: no lesions or blood present

Neck: no lymphadenopathy or JVD

Chest: symmetric, no dullness to percussion. Scattered expiratory wheezes bilaterally, no rales or rhonchi, decreased fremitus throughout.

CV: normal S1, S2, no m/r/g, non-displaced PMI

Ext: no clubbing, cyanosis, or edema

Data Interpretation

DIAGNOSIS 1. LUNG CANCER

History Findings	Physical Exam Findings
Worsening cough and DOE x 3 days	pulse 107/min, respirations 28/min, SpO2: 90%
Blood-tinged sputum	Evidence of respiratory distress
20-lb weight loss and chronic fatigue	Scattered expiratory wheezes
h/o COPD	Decreased fremitus
40 pack year smoking history	

Diagnosis 2. Pneumonia

History Findings	Physical Exam Findings
Worsening cough, fever, DOE x 3 days	pulse 107/min, T 38.3 C, respirations 28/min, SpO2: 90%
Increased sputum production	Evidence of respiratory distress
Intermittent chest tightness, wheezing	Expiratory wheezes on chest exam
h/o pneumonia x 2, COPD	
40 pack year smoking history	

Diagnosis 3. COPD Exacerbation

History Findings	Physical Exam Findings
Worsening cough and DOE x3 days	pulse 107/min, respirations 28/min, SpO2: 90%
Increased sputum production	Evidence of respiratory distress
Increased rescue inhaler use	Expiratory wheezes on chest exam
Intermittent chest tightness, wheezing	Overall decreased tactile fremitus
h/o COPD	Lack of dullness to percussion
40 pack year smoking history	

Diagnostic Studies

CXR

Sputum gram stain & culture

CBC w/ diff

Arterial blood gas

Blood cultures x2

CASE 14: BLOOD IN URINE

Doorway Information

Opening Scenario

Matthew Howe is a 60 year-old man who comes to your office because of intermittent blood in his urine over the past 1 month.

Vital Signs

T 37 C (98.6 F)

BP 150/95 mm Hg

Pulse 62/min

Respirations 14/min

HTN

Examinee Tasks

1. Obtain a pertinent history.

2. Perform a relevant physical examination. Do not perform a pelvic/genital, corneal reflex, or rectal examination.

3. Discuss your impressions and any initial plans with the patient.

4. After leaving the room, complete your patient note.

nephrotic syndrome

UTI

bladder cancer

nephrolithiasis

Communication and Interpersonal Skills Checklist

Fostering the Relationship	Gathering Information	Providing Information
☐ Knocked	☐ Elicited chief complaint	☐ Summarized significant information
☐ Introduced self	☐ Established timeline of patient's CC (chief complaint)	☐ Provided diagnostic impression
☐ Clarified role	☐ Used open-ended question	☐ Justified diagnosis with evidence from encounter
☐ Was properly groomed	☐ Used non-leading questions	☐ Assessed patient's need for additional information
☐ Made eye contact	☐ Used closed-ended questions	☐ Encouraged and answered questions
☐ Maintained appropriate distance	☐ Asked one question at a time	☐ Assessed patient's comprehension of probable illness
☐ Displayed confident manner	☐ Did not use medical jargon	
☐ Showed care and concern	☐ Appropriately used "continuers"	
☐ Was respectful and nonjudgmental	☐ Paraphrased	
☐ Established patient's preferred title	☐ Appropriately used transitions	
☐ Used proper draping	☐ Elicited additional concerns	
☐ Focused on patient	☐ Assessed impact on patient's life	
☐ Did not interrupt patient	☐ Checked for patient understanding	
☐ Maintained appropriate and responsive body language		

Making Decisions	Supporting Emotions
☐ Clearly stated next steps in management	☐ Actively listened and validated patient's expectations
☐ **Counseled** patient	☐ Showed empathy and used appropriate reassurances
☐ Agreed to **mutual plan** of action	☐ Inquired about patient's support system
	☐ Managed the **challenge** (here; patient asked, "is it cancer?")

History and Physical Examination Checklist

HPI

☐ Hematuria   *painless ↑ hematuria*

☐ Duration: 1 month

☐ 3 episodes

☐ Blood present throughout micturition

☐ No pain

☐ Increased urinary frequency

☐ Nocturia 3-4 times per night   *Obs symptoms*

☐ Weak stream

☐ Incomplete voiding

☐ Weight loss

☐ No fever

☐ No chills

☐ No edema

☐ No recent trauma

☐ Sore throat 6 wks ago

☐ No recent travel

PMH

☐ HTN (controlled)

☐ Nephrolithiasis (5 years ago)

☐ No joint pain

☐ No skin rashes

☐ Meds: aspirin and amlodipine

☐ NKDA

Family Hx

☐ Father had prostate cancer

Social Hx

☐ No alcohol, no drugs

☐ Quit smoking

☐ Previous 2 x 30 pack/yr hx of tobacco

☐ Married, monogamous, no hx of STDs

☐ Profession is law, no factory work

☐ No exposure to toxins

Physical Examination

☐ Washed hands prior to examination

☐ Inspected skin

☐ Inspected abdomen

☐ Auscultated abdomen in 4 quadrants

☐ Percussed abdomen in 4 quadrants

☐ Palpated abdomen in 4 quadrants

☐ Examined for costovertebral angle tenderness

☐ Auscultated lungs

☐ Checked for peripheral edema

☐ Checked for peri-orbital edema

Patient Note

History

HPI: 60 y/o man presents with gross hematuria x3 episodes over the past 1 month. The episodes are painless. The blood is seen in the urine throughout the episodes of micturition. ROS is also notable for urinary frequency, nocturia, weak stream and feeling of incomplete voiding for the past 3-4 mos. He also had a sore throat 6 weeks ago and lost some weight. He denies fever, chills, dysuria, oliguria, edema, uncontrolled hypertension, joint pain or skin rashes. He has a h/o well-controlled HTN. He has a 60-pack-year smoking history but quit 10 years ago. He has no known toxic exposures.

PMH: HTN, 1 episode of nephrolithiasis 5 years ago treated with lithotripsy

Medications: amlodipine, aspirin

Allergies: NKDA

Family Hx: father had prostate cancer

Social Hx: 60-pack-year smoking history, social EtOH, married, monogamous, works as a lawyer

Physical Exam

Vitals: T 98.6 F, 8P 150/95 mm Hg, pulse 62/min, R 14/min

General: comfortable, no acute distress

HEENT: oropharynx without lesions or tonsillar exudates

Chest: clear to auscultation, no wheezes, rales or rhonchi

Abd: +BS x4 quadrants, tympanic to percussion x4 quadrants, non-tender, non-distended, no masses palpated, no organomegaly

Back: no costovertebral angle tenderness

Extremities no peripheral edema

Lymph nodes: no palpable nodes in neck, axilla or groin

Data Interpretation

DIAGNOSIS 1. BLADDER CANCER

History Findings	Physical Exam Findings
Hematuria	No fever
Blood present throughout micturition	No tenderness on palpation or abdominal masses
Increased urinary frequency and urgency	
60 pack year smoking history	

DIAGNOSIS 2. POST-STREPTOCOCCAL GLOMERULONEPHRITIS (GN)

History Findings	Physical Exam Findings
Hematuria	Elevated BP
Hypertension	
Recent pharyngitis	

DIAGNOSIS 3. PROSTATE CANCER

History Findings	Physical Exam Findings
Gross hematuria	No fever
Nocturia	No tenderness on palpation or abdominal masses
Increased urinary frequency and urgency	
Family history of prostate cancer	
Weight loss	

Diagnostic Studies

Prostate exam PSA

Antistreptolysin O titer; complement levels

Urinalysis/urine culture

PSA

CBC with platelet count

BUN, creatinine

PT/INR, PTT

Cytoscopy

CASE 15: PEDIATRIC DIARRHEA

Doorway Information

Opening Scenario

Margaret Swanson is the mother of a 1-year-old son calling your office because he has diarrhea.

Vital Signs

Child is not available for physical exam

Examinee Tasks

1. Obtain a focused history.

2. There is no physical exam in this case.

3. Discuss your initial diagnostic impression and your workup plan with the mother.

4. After leaving the room, complete your patient note on the given form.

Communication and Interpersonal Skills Checklist		
Fostering the Relationship	**Gathering Information**	**Providing Information**
☐ Introduced self ☐ Clarified role ☐ Displayed confident manner ☐ Showed care and concern ☐ Was respectful and nonjudgmental ☐ Established preferred title ☐ Did not interrupt	☐ Elicited chief complaint ☐ Established timeline of patient's CC (chief complaint) ☐ Used open-ended question ☐ Used non-leading questions ☐ Used closed-ended questions ☐ Asked one question at a time ☐ Did not use medical jargon ☐ Appropriately used "continuers" ☐ Paraphrased ☐ Appropriately used transitions ☐ Elicited additional concerns ☐ Assessed impact on patient's life ☐ Checked for understanding	☐ Summarized significant information ☐ Provided diagnostic impression ☐ Justified diagnosis with evidence from encounter ☐ Assessed need for additional information ☐ Encouraged and answered questions ☐ Assessed comprehension of probable illness
Making Decisions	**Supporting Emotions**	
☐ Clearly stated next steps in management ☐ **Counseled** relative ☐ Agreed to **mutual plan** of action	☐ Actively listened and validated expectations ☐ Showed empathy and used appropriate reassurances ☐ Inquired about patient's support system ☐ Managed the **challenge** (here; mother asked, "will he require IV fluids?")	

History and Physical Examination Checklist	

HPI
☐ Diarrhea
  ☐ Watery
  ☐ Duration: 3 days
  ☐ Loose stools
  ☐ Foul smelling
  ☐ Some blood and mucus
  ☐ More diaper changes per day than usual
☐ Vomiting
  ☐ 2 episodes
  ☐ Non-bloody
  ☐ Greenish
☐ Tried oral rehydration therapy
  ☐ Worried child needs IV fluids
☐ Low grade fever
☐ Irritable
☐ Sick contacts: daycare
☐ No Rash
☐ No recent dietary changes
☐ No appetite
☐ Difficulty feeding
	PMH
	☐ No recent illness
	☐ Birth history is unremarkable
	☐ Vaginal delivery at 39 weeks
	☐ Prenatal screenings normal
	☐ Appropriate growth curve
	☐ Age appropriate vaccinations completed
	☐ Recently began to walk and speak a few words
	☐ No hospitalizations or surgery
	☐ Meds: acetaminophen. No prescription meds
	☐ NKDA
	Family Hx
	☐ No similar symptoms with family members
	☐ No siblings
	☐ No significant family history
	Social Hx
	☐ Recent travel to India
	☐ Sick contacts at day care
	☐ Unsure of HIV status

Physical Examination	
No physical exam	

Patient Note

History

HPI: 1 y/o boy with 3-day history of diarrhea and episodes of non- bloody, greenish vomitus. Mother describes stools as watery, loose, and foul-smelling. Once or twice there was some blood and mucus in the stool. Child is on oral rehydration solution. Child has had a low-grade fever and has been extremely irritable. The child's playmates at the day care have also become ill, though no one in the family is affected. There is no rash or high fever. Family did recently travel to India to visit relatives. The child was healthy and active prior to the onset of symptoms.

PMH: none

Birth Hx: unremarkable; mother had normal spontaneous vaginal delivery at 39 wks. Mother had unremarkable pre-natal course. All prenatal evaluations were reportedly normal

Allergies: NKDA

Medications: pediatric acetaminophen as needed

Social Hx: lives at home with his parents, no siblings

Family Hx: unremarkable

Immunization hx: up-to-date according to age

Physical Exam

There is no physical examination in this case.

Data Interpretation

DIAGNOSIS 1. ACUTE BACTERIAL GASTROENTERITIS

History Findings	Physical Exam Findings
Irritability	No physical exam
Bloody diarrhea	
Recent travel history	
Vomiting	
Fever	
Sick contacts	

Diagnosis 2. Acute Viral Gastroenteritis

History Findings	Physical Exam Findings
Irritability	No physical exam
Watery diarrhea	
Low-grade fever	
Vomiting	
Daycare exposure	

Diagnosis 3. Giardiasis

History Findings	Physical Exam Findings
Irritability	No physical exam
Watery diarrhea	
Foul-smelling diarrhea	
Recent travel history	
Vomiting	

Diagnostic Studies

Physical exam of patient

CBC with differential

Serum electrolytes

Stool culture, fecal leucocytes

Stool for ova and parasites

Rotavirus enzyme immunoassay

Fecal leukocytes

CASE 16: DIZZINESS

Doorway Information

Opening Scenario

Connie Thomas is a 43-year-old woman who comes to your office complaining of dizziness.

Vital Signs

T 37.0 C (98.6 F)

BP 128/84 mm Hg   ∨SS

Pulse 66/min

Respirations 14/min

Examinee Tasks

1. Obtain a focused history.

2. Perform a relevant physical exam. Do not perform rectal, pelvic, genitourinary, female breast, or corneal reflex exam.

3. Discuss your initial diagnostic impression and your workup plan with the patient.

4. After leaving the room, complete your Patient Note on the given form.

Communication and Interpersonal Skills Checklist

Fostering the Relationship	Gathering Information	Providing Information
☐ Knocked	☐ Elicited chief complaint	☐ Summarized significant information
☐ Introduced self	☐ Established timeline of patient's CC (chief complaint)	☐ Provided diagnostic impression
☐ Clarified role	☐ Used open-ended question	☐ Justified diagnosis with evidence from encounter
☐ Was properly groomed	☐ Used non-leading questions	☐ Assessed patient's need for additional information
☐ Made eye contact	☐ Used closed-ended questions	☐ Encouraged and answered questions
☐ Maintained appropriate distance	☐ Asked one question at a time	☐ Assessed patient's comprehension of probable illness
☐ Displayed confident manner	☐ Did not use medical jargon	
☐ Showed care and concern	☐ Appropriately used "continuers"	
☐ Was respectful and nonjudgmental	☐ Paraphrased	
☐ Established patient's preferred title	☐ Appropriately used transitions	
☐ Used proper draping	☐ Elicited additional concerns	
☐ Focused on patient	☐ Assessed impact on patient's life	
☐ Did not interrupt patient	☐ Checked for patient understanding	
☐ Maintained appropriate and responsive body language		

Making Decisions	Supporting Emotions
☐ Clearly stated next steps in management	☐ Actively listened and validated patient's expectations
☐ **Counseled** patient	☐ Showed empathy and used appropriate reassurances
☐ Agreed to **mutual plan** of action	☐ Inquired about patient's support system
	☐ Managed the **challenge** (here; patient has difficulty understanding you)

Meniers disease

History and Physical Examination Checklist

HPI
- ☐ Episodic dizziness
- ☐ Duration: 6 mos
- ☐ Last episode 1 week ago
- ☐ Unsteady on feet
- ☐ Room spinning
- ☐ Spell duration: 20 minutes
- ☐ No precipitating factor
- ☐ Relieved by lying still
- ☐ Aggravated by positional changes
- ☐ + nausea
- ☐ + vomiting
- ☐ Fluctuating hearing loss
  - ☐ Difficulty understanding speech
  - ☐ Left ear > right
  - ☐ Sensation of fullness in the ear
  - ☐ Low pitched buzz heard predominately in left ear
- ☐ No fever
- ☐ No chills
- ☐ No weakness
- ☐ No sensory changes
- ☐ No visual changes
- ☐ No headache
- ☐ No syncope

PMH
- ☐ No similar illness
- ☐ No history of head trauma
- ☐ History of HTN
- ☐ No hospitalizations or surgery
- ☐ Meds: atenolol and aspirin
- ☐ NKDA

Family Hx
- ☐ Father hx of stroke and HTN
- ☐ Mother hx of high cholesterol

Social Hx
- ☐ No Tobacco use
- ☐ No alcohol use
- ☐ No recreational drug use
- ☐ Regular exercise
- ☐ On a healthy diet
- ☐ Single, lives alone
- ☐ Works as a web designer

Physical Examination

- ☐ Washed hands prior to examination
- ☐ Performed inspection of head
- ☐ Performed fundoscopic exam
- ☐ Performed pupillary reflex
- ☐ Performed external ear and otoscopic exams
- ☐ Performed Weber's test
  - ☐ Sounds lateralized to the right
- ☐ Performed Rinne's test
  - ☐ Air conduction > bone conduction bilaterally
- ☐ Examined CN II–XII
- ☐ Assessed motor strength bilaterally
- ☐ Examined DTRs
- ☐ Assessed 2 modalities of sensation (light, sharp/dull)
- ☐ Assessed cerebellar function with finger-to-nose or rapid alternating movements
- ☐ Performed Romberg test
  - ☐ Negative

meniere's

Patient Note

History

HPI: 43 y/o woman complains of dizziness for past 6 mos with most recent episode occurring 1 week ago. There is no clear precipitant. The dizziness is described as the room spinning and gait unsteadiness. Episodes last from 20 minutes to a few hours and are associated with fluctuating loss of hearing, fullness and a buzzing sound all in the left ear, and sometimes nausea and vomiting. Dizziness is relieved by lying still; positional changes seem to make it worse. ROS negative for fever, chills, weakness, sensory changes, visual changes, headache, syncope

PMH: HTN, no history of head trauma

Allergies: denies

Meds: aspirin, atenolol

FH: father had a stroke, mother has HTN, HLD

SH: denies smoking, illicit drug use, and heavy EtOH use. Single, lives alone, and works as web designer

Physical Examination

BP 128/84 mm Hg, pulse 66/min, T 37.0 C, Respirations 14/min

Gen: appears comfortable and NAD, speech is normal

HEENT: Normocephalic, atraumatic, no papilledema or optic disc blurring on fundoscopy, PEERLA, EOMI, TM seen; no erythema, polyps or exudates; Weber test: lateralizes to R side; Rinne test: AC > BC bilaterally

Neuro: CN II–XII intact, motor: 5/5 b/l, DTR: 2+ bilaterally: l sensory system grossly intact, negative Romberg test, no intention tremor/dysmetria/gait abnormalities

Data Interpretation

DIAGNOSIS 1. MENIERE'S DISEASE

History Findings	Physical Exam Findings
Episodic vertigo	Weber and Rinne tests suggest sensorineural hearing loss
Lasts from 20 min to few hrs	Normal speech pattern
Tinnitus and aural fullness	CN II–XII intact
Fluctuating hearing loss	Motor: 5/5 bilaterally
Ataxia during epiodes	Sensory intact
Nausea and vomiting	

DIAGNOSIS 2. BENIGN PAROXYSMAL POSITIONAL VERTIGO

History Findings	Physical Exam Findings
Episodic vertigo worse with positional changes	CN II–XII intact
Ataxia during episodes	Motor: 5/5 bilaterally
Nausea, vomiting	Sensory intact

DIAGNOSIS 3. ACOUSTIC NEUROMA

History Findings	Physical Exam Findings
Vertigo was gradual in onset 6 mos ago	Weber and Rinne tests suggest sensori-neural hearing loss
Tinnitus and aural fullness	
Hearing loss	
Ataxia during episodes	

Diagnostic Studies

Head MRI

Dix-Hallpike test

Audiogram

head MRI
audiology
Dix-Hallpike

CASE 17: DIFFICULTY SWALLOWING

Doorway Information

Opening Scenario

Gary Schwartz is a 52-year-old man who presents to your office complaining of difficulty swallowing. *dysphagia*

Vital Signs

T 37.3 C (99.1 F)

BP 148/78 mm Hg

Pulse 74/min

Respirations 16/min

Examinee Tasks

1. Obtain a focused history.

2. Perform a relevant physical exam. Do not perform rectal, pelvic, genitourinary, or corneal reflex exam.

3. Discuss your initial diagnostic impression and your workup plan with the patient.

4. After leaving the room, complete your Patient Note on the given form.

Communication and Interpersonal Skills Checklist

Fostering the Relationship

- ☐ Knocked
- ☐ Introduced self
- ☐ Clarified role
- ☐ Was properly groomed
- ☐ Made eye contact
- ☐ Maintained appropriate distance
- ☐ Displayed confident manner
- ☐ Showed care and concern
- ☐ Was respectful and nonjudgmental
- ☐ Established patient's preferred title
- ☐ Used proper draping
- ☐ Focused on patient
- ☐ Did not interrupt patient
- ☐ Maintained appropriate and responsive body language

Gathering Information

- ☐ Elicited chief complaint
- ☐ Established timeline of patient's CC (chief complaint)
- ☐ Used open-ended question
- ☐ Used non-leading questions
- ☐ Used closed-ended questions
- ☐ Asked one question at a time
- ☐ Did not use medical jargon
- ☐ Appropriately used "continuers"
- ☐ Paraphrased
- ☐ Appropriately used transitions
- ☐ Elicited additional concerns
- ☐ Assessed impact on patient's life
- ☐ Checked for patient understanding

Providing Information

- ☐ Summarized significant information
- ☐ Provided diagnostic impression
- ☐ Justified diagnosis with evidence from encounter
- ☐ Assessed patient's need for additional information
- ☐ Encouraged and answered questions
- ☐ Assessed patient's comprehension of probable illness

Making Decisions

- ☐ Clearly stated next steps in management
- ☐ **Counseled** patient
- ☐ Agreed to **mutual plan** of action

Supporting Emotions

- ☐ Actively listened and validated patient's expectations
- ☐ Showed empathy and used appropriate reassurances
- ☐ Inquired about patient's support system
- ☐ Managed the **challenge** (here; patient has difficulty understanding you)

*w/u   EGD
CT chest /abd
CBC
lytes*

History and Physical Examination Checklist

HPI

- ☐ Difficulty swallowing
- ☐ Duration: 1 Month *obs mechanical*
- ☐ Affects (solids) *~ obs mechanical*
- ☐ Sensation of food stuck in throat
- ☐ No problem with liquids or semi-solids
- ☐ Progressively worse
  - ☐ Initially could compensate by chewing longer
- ☐ Occasional food regurgitation
- ☐ No associated pain
- ☐ No alleviating or aggravating factors
- ☐ Fatigue
- ☐ Bad breath
- ☐ Weight loss
  - ☐ 15 lbs
  - ☐ Unintentional
- ☐ No nausea
- ☐ No vomiting
- ☐ No diarrhea
- ☐ No blood in stool
- ☐ No fever
- ☐ No chills
- ☐ No SOB

PMH

- ☐ Hx of GERD
- ☐ Treated with antacids
- ☐ No hospitalizations or surgery
- ☐ Meds: aspirin
- ☐ NKDA

Family Hx

- ☐ Father died of lung cancer
- ☐ Mother hx of CAD and HTN

Social Hx

- ☐ Smoked 30 pack yrs
- ☐ Drinks 3-4 glasses of wine/night
- ☐ No recreational drug use
- ☐ Married with 3 children
- ☐ Works as an accountant

Physical Examination

*- esophageal cancer
adeno vs SCC
- esophageal web
- stricture*

- ☐ Washed hands prior to examination
- ☐ Inspected oropharynx
- ☐ Inspected thyroid gland
- ☐ Palpated thyroid gland
- ☐ Palpated neck for lymphadenopathy
- ☐ Checked for axillary lymphadenopathy
- ☐ Auscultated abdomen
- ☐ Listened for bowel sounds in 4 quadrants
- ☐ Percussed abdomen in 4 quadrants
- ☐ Palpated abdomen in 4 quadrants

Patient Note

History

HPI: 52 y/o man c/o difficulty swallowing solid foods, though not liquids or semisolid foods, for the past 1 month. The difficulty swallowing is described as "food getting stuck in his chest" and has progressively worsened. At first, he was able to compensate by chewing his food for longer than usual, but now it has progressed to the point where he has trouble with most of his meals and reports occasional regurgitation of food. He says nothing makes the symptoms better or worse other than avoiding meats and breads. ROS also notable for bad breath that is unrelieved with breath mints, 15 pound weight loss, and mild fatigue. The patient denies nausea, vomiting, diarrhea, blood in his stool, fevers, chills, or shortness of breath. He has a h/o GERD treated with OTC medication. He has a 30 year pack history of smoking and drinks 3-4 glasses of wine at night.

PMH: GERD

Allergies: NKDA

Medications: aspirin and Tums as needed

Family Hx: Father died of lung cancer, mother has CAD and HTN

Social Hx: smoking and EtOH history as above, and he denies use of illicit drugs. He is married with 3 children and works as an accountant.

Physical Exam

T 99.1 F, BP 148/78 mm Hg, pulse 74/min, respirations 16/min

General: appears older than stated age and is thin, but in no acute distress

HEENT: oropharynx without lesions or tonsillar exudates, good dentition

Neck: no thyromegaly or nodules, no cervical or supraclavicular lymphadenopathy

Axilla: no palpable lymphadenopathy

CV: RRR, normal S1, S2, no murmurs, rubs, or gallops

Chest: clear to auscultation, no wheezes, rales or rhonchi

Abd: +BS x4 quadrants, tympanic to percussion x4 quadrants, non-tender, non-distended, no masses or organomegaly

Extremities: no cyanosis, clubbing or edema

Data Interpretation

DIAGNOSIS 1. ESOPHAGEAL CARCINOMA

History Findings	Physical Exam Findings
Progressive dysphagia to solids	Appears older than stated age and thin
h/o GERD	
30 pack year smoking history	
Daily EtOH use	
15 lb weight loss	

DIAGNOSIS 2. ESOPHAGEAL STRICTURE

History Findings	Physical Exam Findings
Dysphagia	
h/o GERD	
Regurgitation of food	
Weight loss	

DIAGNOSIS 3. ACHALASIA

History Findings	Physical Exam Findings
Dysphagia	Thin-appearing
Regurgitation of food	
15 lb weight loss	

Diagnostic Studies

CBC

Chest CT

Barium esophagram — Barium swallow

Esophagogastroduodenoscopy (EGD)

Esophageal manometry — manometry

CASE 18: SHORTNESS OF BREATH

Doorway Information

Opening Scenario

Mario Hernandez is a 60-year-old man who presents to the ER with shortness of breath.

Vital Signs

T 37 C (98.6 F)

BP 170/95 mm Hg   *— HTN*

Pulse 96/min

Respirations 24/min

Oxygen saturation: 90% on room air   *hypoxic*

Examinee Tasks

1. Obtain a focused history.

2. Perform a relevant physical exam. Do not perform rectal, pelvic, genitourinary, or corneal reflex exam.

3. Discuss your initial diagnostic impression and your workup plan with the patient.

4. After leaving the room, complete your Patient Note on the given form.

Communication and Interpersonal Skills Checklist		
Fostering the Relationship	**Gathering Information**	**Providing Information**
☐ Knocked ☐ Introduced self ☐ Clarified role ☐ Was properly groomed ☐ Made eye contact ☐ Maintained appropriate distance ☐ Displayed confident manner ☐ Showed care and concern ☐ Was respectful and nonjudgmental ☐ Established patient's preferred title ☐ Used proper draping ☐ Focused on patient ☐ Did not interrupt patient ☐ Maintained appropriate and responsive body language	☐ Elicited chief complaint ☐ Established timeline of patient's CC (chief complaint) ☐ Used open-ended question ☐ Used non-leading questions ☐ Used closed-ended questions ☐ Asked one question at a time ☐ Did not use medical jargon ☐ Appropriately used "continuers" ☐ Paraphrased ☐ Appropriately used transitions ☐ Elicited additional concerns ☐ Assessed impact on patient's life ☐ Checked for patient understanding	☐ Summarized significant information ☐ Provided diagnostic impression ☐ Justified diagnosis with evidence from encounter ☐ Assessed patient's need for additional information ☐ Encouraged and answered questions ☐ Assessed patient's comprehension of probable illness
Making Decisions	**Supporting Emotions**	
☐ Clearly stated next steps in management ☐ **Counseled** patient ☐ Agreed to **mutual plan** of action	☐ Actively listened and validated patient's expectations ☐ Showed empathy and used appropriate reassurances ☐ Inquired about patient's support system ☐ Managed the **challenge** (here; patient says," Doc, I can't breathe?")	

History and Physical Examination Checklist

HPI

☐ Repeated episodes of shortness of breath

☐ Duration: 3 mos

☐ Occurs with exertion

☐ Progressively worse

    ☐ Can no longer climb stairs

    ☐ SOB after walking 1 city block

☐ Mild cough   *Sarcoid?*

    ☐ Occasionally productive

    ☐ Pink tinged, frothy sputum

☐ Low grade fever

☐ Symptoms worse when he lies down   *CHF*

    ☐ Wakes up gasping for air when lying flat

    ☐ Sleeps in a recliner

☐ Symptoms improve when sitting upright

☐ Swollen legs

☐ Weight gain

    ☐ 10 lbs

    ☐ Over 1 month

    ☐ No appetite

☐ No chest pain

☐ No chills

☐ No diaphoresis

☐ No wheezing

☐ No muscle or joint aches

☐ No urinary symptoms

☐ No nausea

☐ No vomiting or diarrhea

PMH

☐ Hx of type 2 diabetes mellitus, HTN, and hyperlipidemia

☐ Meds: hydrochlorothiazide, simvastatin, and metformin

☐ No hx of surgery

☐ NKDA

Family Hx

☐ Father died of a heart attack

☐ Age 50

☐ Brother with hx of HTN and diabetes

Social Hx

☐ Smoker: 40 pack yrs

☐ Drinks socially

☐ Cocaine use for past 4 mos

☐ Married with 4 children

☐ Retired factory worker

Physical Examination

☐ Washed hands prior to examination

☐ Performed inspection of chest

☐ Performed percussion of lungs bilaterally

☐ Palpated for tactile fremitus bilaterally

☐ Auscultated lungs

    ☐ Coughs when asked to breathe deeply or expire fully

    ☐ rales 1/3 up from the lung bases

    ☐ no wheezes

    ☐ no rhonchi

☐ Examined for JVD

    ☐ JVD halfway to the angle of the jaw

☐ Palpated PMI

    ☐ Laterally displaced PMI

☐ Auscultated heart in 4 areas

☐ Examined extremeties for edema

    ☐ 2+ pitting edema

☐ Assessed for hepatojugular reflex

    ☐ + hepatojugular reflex

Patient Note

History

HPI: 60 y/o man presents to the ER with dyspnea on exertion that is progressively worsening for the past 2-3 mos. He has trouble walking up one flight of stairs and becomes very SOB after ambulating less than one city block. He has orthopnea to the point where he now sleeps in a recliner and also reports paroxysmal nocturnal dyspnea. He has a 10 pound weight gain and swelling of his lower extremities. ROS also notable for productive cough of pink, frothy sputum and intermittent low grade fever for the past 2 weeks. He denies chest pain, fever, shaking chills, wheezing, muscle or joint aches, urinary symptoms, nausea, vomiting or diarrhea. He is a smoker with a 40 pack year history and uses cocaine.

PMHx: DM2, HTN, HLD, no surgeries

Medications: simvastatin, metformin, hydrochlorothiazide. NKDA

Family Hx: father died of MI in his 50s, brother has HTN and DM2

Physical Exam

T 98.6 F, BP 170/95 mm Hg, pulse 96/min, respirations 24/min, SaO$_2$: 90% on room air

General: appears to be in moderate respiratory distress, coughing often

Chest: symmetrical, normal percussion, normal tactile fremitus, rales 1/3 up from the lung bases, no wheezes or rhonchi

CVS: RRR, normal S1, S2, and +S3 gallop, no murmurs/rubs, PMI is laterally displaced, +JVD halfway to angle of jaw, +hepatojugular reflex

Extremities: 2+ LE pitting edema

Data Interpretation

DIAGNOSIS 1. CONGESTIVE HEART FAILURE/ISCHEMIC CARDIOMYOPATHY

History Findings	Physical Exam Findings
Progressive DOE	SpO2: 90%, respiratory distress
Orthopnea, paroxysmal dyspnea	Rales on lung exam
Leg swelling	JVD, S3 gallop
h/o HTN, DM2, HLD	+hepatojugular reflex
h/o heavy cigarette smoking	2+ LE pitting edema
FH heart disease	

DIAGNOSIS 2. NON-ISCHEMIC CARDIOMYOPATHY

History Findings	Physical Exam Findings
Progressive DOE	SpO2: 90%, respiratory distress
Orthopnea, paroxysmal dyspnea	Rales on lung exam
LE swelling	JVD, S3 gallop
h/o fevers	+hepatojugular reflex
h/o cocaine use, social EtOH	2+ LE pitting edema

Diagnostic Studies

EKG

Chest x-ray

Lipid profile

Echocardiogram

Troponin, CK-MB

BNP

CBC

Urine toxicology

CASE 19: ADULT NOSEBLEED

Doorway Information

Opening Scenario

Kevin Green is a 45-year-old man who presents to your office with chronic nose-bleeds.

Vital Signs

T 36.8°C (98.2°F)

BP 110/80 mm Hg

Pulse 88/min regular

Respirations 18/min

Examinee Tasks

1. Obtain a focused history.

2. Perform a relevant physical exam. Do not perform rectal, pelvic, genitourinary, or corneal reflex exams.

3. Discuss your initial diagnostic impression and your workup plan with the patient.

4. After leaving the room, complete your Patient Note on the given form.

Communication and Interpersonal Skills Checklist		
Fostering the Relationship	**Gathering Information**	**Providing Information**
☐ Knocked ☐ Introduced self ☐ Clarified role ☐ Was properly groomed ☐ Made eye contact ☐ Maintained appropriate distance ☐ Displayed confident manner ☐ Showed care and concern ☐ Was respectful and nonjudgmental ☐ Established patient's preferred title ☐ Used proper draping ☐ Focused on patient ☐ Did not interrupt patient ☐ Maintained appropriate and responsive body language	☐ Elicited chief complaint ☐ Established timeline of patient's CC (chief complaint) ☐ Used open-ended question ☐ Used non-leading questions ☐ Used closed-ended questions ☐ Asked one question at a time ☐ Did not use medical jargon ☐ Appropriately used "continuers" ☐ Paraphrased ☐ Appropriately used transitions ☐ Elicited additional concerns ☐ Assessed impact on patient's life ☐ Checked for patient understanding	☐ Summarized significant information ☐ Provided diagnostic impression ☐ Justified diagnosis with evidence from encounter ☐ Assessed patient's need for additional information ☐ Encouraged and answered questions ☐ Assessed patient's comprehension of probable illness
Making Decisions		**Supporting Emotions**
☐ Clearly stated next steps in management ☐ **Counseled** patient ☐ Agreed to **mutual plan** of action		☐ Actively listened and validated patient's expectations ☐ Showed empathy and used appropriate reassurances ☐ Inquired about patient's support system ☐ Managed the **challenge** (here; patient asked, "Is it serious?")

- Nasopharyngeal Carcinoma
- Polyp?
- Med side effect
- Yikes
- ITP
- Nutritional deficiency
- liver failure

History and Physical Examination Checklist	
HPI	**PMH**

HPI

- ☐ Epistaxis
- ☐ Duration: 3 mos
- ☐ Intermittent
  - ☐ Occurs 1-2 times per week
- ☐ Bleed mostly from left nostril
- ☐ Started after a bad cold
  - ☐ Continued after the cold resolved
- ☐ Quantity of blood
  - ☐ Variable
  - ☐ Severe bleeding twice
- ☐ Self-treatment with tissues up his nose
- ☐ Aggravated by
  - ☐ Sneezing
  - ☐ Blowing his nose

- ☐ Nothing makes it better
- ☐ No other nasal discharge
- ☐ No recent trauma to nose
- ☐ + bruising easily
- ☐ 10 lbs weight gain
  - ☐ Over 6 mos
  - ☐ Poor diet
    - ☐ Fast food
    - ☐ No vegetables
    - ☐ No fruits
- ☐ Decreased appetite
- ☐ No fever
- ☐ No chills
- ☐ No sore throat
- ☐ No headache
- ☐ No GI bleeding
- ☐ No gingival bleeding
- ☐ Itchy skin
  - ☐ >6 mos

Cholestasis (handwritten)

PMH

- ☐ No similar nose prior to these 3 mos
- ☐ No HTN
- ☐ + degenerative joint disease of knee
- ☐ Treated with acetaminophen   *Max dose* (handwritten)
  - ☐ 8 tablets per day
- ☐ No hospitalizations or surgery
- ☐ No history of blood transfusions
- ☐ Meds: no prescription meds
- ☐ NKDA

Family Hx

- ☐ No family history of bleeding disorders or blood clots
- ☐ Not been around anyone sick recently
- ☐ Family history of heavy drinking
- ☐ Mother died age late 50s

Social Hx

- ☐ Single
- ☐ Sexually active
- ☐ With women
- ☐ Unsure of HIV status
- ☐ No recreational drug use
- ☐ Previous 2 x 25 pack/yr hx of tobacco
- ☐ Drinks 5 shots of bourbon daily
- ☐ Unemployed
- ☐ Previously a construction worker

Physical Examination	

- ☐ Washed hands prior to examination
- ☐ Inspected skin for
  - ☐ Jaundice (+)
  - ☐ Multiple ecchymoses on extremities and trunk (+)
  - ☐ Palmar erythema (−)
  - ☐ spider angiomata (−)
- ☐ Inspected eye for scleral icterus
  - ☐ non-injected
  - ☐ (+) scleral icterus
- ☐ Inspected nares
- ☐ Inspected oropharynx
- ☐ Inspected abdomen
- ☐ Auscultated abdomen
  - ☐ +BS in all 4 quadrants

- ☐ Percussed abdomen
- ☐ Palpated abdomen
  - ☐ Soft and non-tender to palpation
- ☐ Assessed abdomen for ascites
  - ☐ No fluid wave
- ☐ Assessed liver and spleen size
  - ☐ No obvious organomegaly
- ☐ Assessed for asterixis
  - ☐ No flapping tremor
  - ☐ AAO x 3
- ☐ Examined extremities for edema
  - ☐ No edema

[handwritten notes at top of page:] AST ALT ALP GTT Tbili. direct bili. INR 77 PTT albumin lytes (Na, Cr, BUN) CBC w/ diff HBV HCV labs imaging U/S RUQ abd U/S EGD varices vitamin C acetaminophen liver

Patient Note

History

HPI: 45 y/o man presents to the office complaining of epistaxis for the past 3 mos that began after a URI. The bleeds occur in the left nostril, happen 1-2 x per week, and usually self-resolve, but there were 2 episodes where the bleeding was especially heavy. Placing tissue in the nostril usually slows down the bleeding, and sneezing or blowing the nose forcefully makes it worse. ROS also notable for easy bruising and an unintentional 10 lb weight gain, decreased appetite, and itchy skin for more than 6 months.. ROS negative for trauma, history of frequent nosebleeds in the past, fevers or chills, sore throat, headache, GI bleeding, gingival bleeding, high BP, family history of bleeding disorder or blood clots. He takes about 8 acetaminophen a day for DJD of the knees. He also drinks 5 shots of bourbon daily. He has a poor diet lacking in fruits and vegetables.

[handwritten: - heavy drinking - tylenol - 4 sex partners]

PMHx: DJD of the knees

Allergies: NKDA

Meds: Tylenol

SHx: 5 shots of bourbon daily,2 packs of cigarettes per day for 25 yrs, no other illicit drugs, single, sexually active with women, unemployed but used to work in construction.

FHx: Mother was a heavy drinker, died in her late 50s.

Physical Exam

BP 110/80 mm Hg, pulse 88/min, T 36.8 C, respirations 18/min

Gen: NAD, slightly disheveled appearance, skin is jaundiced

HEENT: Sclera are not injected, but there is icterus, PERRLA, EOMI, left nostril shows crusted blood but no active bleeding, right nostril is normal. Oropharynx shows poor dentition, but no lesions.

Abd: +BS x4 quadrants, dullness to percussion, soft and non-tender, no organomegaly

Extremities: thin and without edema

Skin: multiple ecchymoses on extremities and trunk, no palmar erythema or spider angiomata

Neuro: AAOx3, no flapping tremor

Data Interpretation

DIAGNOSIS 1. HEPATIC FAILURE

History Findings	Physical Exam Findings
Recurrent epistaxis	Evidence of recent nosebleed
2 episodes of heavy bleeding	Jaundice, scleral icterus
Easy bruising, itchy skin	Multiple bruises
Weight gain, decreased appetite	Dullness to percussion
Excessive acetaminophen use	
Heavy drinking history	
Sexually active with multiple women	

Diagnosis 2. Nutritional deficiency/vitamin C or K deficiency

History Findings	Physical Exam Findings
Recurrent epistaxis	Evidence of recent nosebleed
2 episodes of heavy bleeding	Poor dentition
Easy bruising	Multiple bruises
Poor diet	Thin extremities
Heavy drinking	

Diagnosis 3. Thrombocytopenia (ITP, splenic sequestration, leukemia)

History Findings	Physical Exam Findings
Recurrent epistaxis	Evidence of recent nosebleed
2 episodes of heavy bleeding	Multiple bruises
Easy bruising	

Diagnostic Studies

CBC with differential and platelet count

Hepatic function panel (AST, ALT, alk phos, total bilirubin (direct and indirect), total protein, albumin)

PT/INR, PTT, fibrinogen, D-Dimer, Bleeding time

Acetaminophen level

Vitamin C level

Abdominal U/S

CASE 20: ADOLESCENT WEIGHT LOSS

Doorway Information

Opening Scenario

Mr. Wright comes to your clinic to discuss his 14-year-old granddaughter, Amy, who is losing weight.

Vital Signs

N/A

Examinee Tasks

1. Obtain a focused history.

2. You will not be required to perform a physical exam in this case.

3. Discuss your initial diagnostic impression and your workup plan with the patient.

4. After leaving the room, complete your Patient Note on the given form.

Communication and Interpersonal Skills Checklist		
Fostering the Relationship	**Gathering Information**	**Providing Information**
☐ Knocked ☐ Introduced self ☐ Clarified role ☐ Was properly groomed ☐ Made eye contact ☐ Maintained appropriate distance ☐ Displayed confident manner ☐ Showed care and concern ☐ Was respectful and nonjudgmental ☐ Established preferred title ☐ Focused on patient ☐ Did not interrupt ☐ Maintained appropriate and responsive body language	☐ Elicited chief complaint ☐ Established timeline of patient's CC (chief complaint) ☐ Used open-ended question ☐ Used non-leading questions ☐ Used closed-ended questions ☐ Asked one question at a time ☐ Did not use medical jargon ☐ Appropriately used "continuers" ☐ Paraphrased ☐ Appropriately used transitions ☐ Elicited additional concerns ☐ Assessed impact on patient's life ☐ Checked for understanding	☐ Summarized significant information ☐ Provided diagnostic impression ☐ Justified diagnosis with evidence from encounter ☐ Assessed need for additional information ☐ Encouraged and answered questions ☐ Assessed comprehension of probable illness
Making Decisions	**Supporting Emotions**	
☐ Clearly stated next steps in management ☐ **Counseled** relative ☐ Agreed to **mutual plan** of action	☐ Actively listened and validated expectations ☐ Showed empathy and used appropriate reassurances ☐ Inquired about patient's support system ☐ Managed the **challenge** (here; grandfather asked, "What can I do?")	

History and Physical Examination Checklist

HPI

- ☐ Weight loss
  - ☐ 25 lbs lost
  - ☐ Over 6 mos
  - ☐ Weight 80 lbs
  - ☐ Height 5'3
- ☐ Patient lacks concern about weight loss
  - ☐ Thinks weight is normal
- ☐ Excessive exercise
  - ☐ Hundreds of sit ups each night
  - ☐ Works out with gymnastics team during the week
  - ☐ Works out alone on the weekend
  - ☐ Goal to be on the Olympic team
- ☐ Caloric intake not clear to grandfather
  - ☐ Claims to like food
  - ☐ Pushes about food on her plate at meals
  - ☐ Snacks on carrots and lettuce
- ☐ Menarche at age 12
- ☐ Amenorrhea
  - ☐ >12 mos
- ☐ Heat intolerance
- ☐ Increased sweating
- ☐ Palpitations
  - ☐ Especially after working out
- ☐ Drinks a lot of ice cold water
  - ☐ To cleanse her system
- ☐ No fever
- ☐ No chills
- ☐ No headache
- ☐ No nausea
- ☐ No vomiting
- ☐ No diarrhea
- ☐ No dysuria
- ☐ No easy bruising or bleeding

PMH

- ☐ No history of depression
- ☐ Appears to have recovered from death of mother
- ☐ Emergency appendectomy at age 6
- ☐ Meds: No prescription meds
- ☐ Grandfather discovered laxatives in her room
- ☐ NKDA

Family Hx

- ☐ Mother with history of depression
- ☐ Mother deceased
- ☐ Accident with drunk driver
- ☐ 1 yr ago
- ☐ Grandfather has history of anxiety

Social Hx

- ☐ Lives with grandfather since mother's death
- ☐ Good performance in school
- ☐ Participates in sports
- ☐ Gymnastics
- ☐ Pressure from coach on weight
- ☐ Not sexually active
- ☐ No drug use
- ☐ No smoking
- ☐ No alcohol

MSE
lytes, EKG
hospitalization?
Utox

TSH T4
LH FSH

Physical Examination

No physical exam

Patient Note

History

HPI: 14 y/o girl shows 25 lb weight loss over 6 mos. Her grandfather states that she was always thin but now he is concerned. She talks about her love of food but doesn't eat much. Grandfather is not sure about how much she actually eats. She is a gymnast and exercises excessively. She is currently 5 feet 3 inches and 80 lbs, but pt still believes she is overweight. Has associated heat intolerance, sweats, palpitations, especially after working out, and sometimes excessive water intake. Denies fevers, chills, headaches, nausea, vomiting, diarrhea, dysuria, easy bruising, and bleeding. No menstrual period in past year, despite menarche at age 12. Grandfather found bottles of laxatives in her room.

PMHx: emergency appendectomy at age 6

Meds: no Rx, laxatives

Allergies: NKDA

SHx: does well in school; does not drink, smoke, or use illicit drugs. Not sexually active.

FHx: notable for depression in mother, grandfather has anxiety

Physical Examination

There is no physical examination in this case.

Data Interpretation

DIAGNOSIS 1. ANOREXIA NERVOSA

History Findings	Physical Exam Findings
25 lb weight loss	No physical exam
Excessive exercising	
Distorted body image	
Amenorrhea	
Laxative use	

DIAGNOSIS 2. HYPERTHYROIDISM

History Findings	Physical Exam Findings
25 lb weight loss	No physical exam
Amenorrhea	
Palpitations	
Heat intolerance	

DIAGNOSIS 3. BULIMIA

History Findings	Physical Exam Findings
Excessive exercising	No physical exam
Laxative use	
Preoccupation with body weight	

Diagnostic Studies

Physical exam   MSE

TSH, free T3, free T4

FSH, LH, prolactin

BUN, creatinine, electrolytes (Na, K, Cl, HCO3, Ca, Mg, phos)

Total protein, albumin , ESR

EKG

CASE 21: PEDIATRIC VOMITING AND DIARRHEA

> ## Doorway Information
>
> ## Opening Scenario
>
> Lilian James is an 18-month-old girl whose mother calls the physician about the child's vomiting and diarrhea for the past 2 days.
>
> ## Vital Signs
>
> There are no vital signs taken in this case.
>
> ## Examinee Tasks
>
> 1. Obtain a focused history.
>
> 2. You will not be required to perform a physical exam in this case.
>
> 3. Discuss your initial diagnostic impression and your workup plan with the patient.
>
> 4. After leaving the room, complete your Patient Note on the given form.

Communication and Interpersonal Skills Checklist		
Fostering the Relationship	**Gathering Information**	**Providing Information**
☐ Introduced self ☐ Clarified role ☐ Displayed confident manner ☐ Showed care and concern ☐ Was respectful and nonjudgmental ☐ Established preferred title ☐ Did not interrupt	☐ Elicited chief complaint ☐ Established timeline of patient's CC (chief complaint) ☐ Used open-ended question ☐ Used non-leading questions ☐ Used closed-ended questions ☐ Asked one question at a time ☐ Did not use medical jargon ☐ Appropriately used "continuers" ☐ Paraphrased ☐ Appropriately used transitions ☐ Elicited additional concerns ☐ Assessed impact on patient's life ☐ Checked for patient understanding	☐ Summarized significant information ☐ Provided diagnostic impression ☐ Justified diagnosis with evidence from encounter ☐ Assessed need for additional information ☐ Encouraged and answered questions ☐ Assessed comprehension of probable illness
Making Decisions	**Supporting Emotions**	
☐ Clearly stated next steps in management ☐ **Counseled** relative ☐ Agreed to **mutual plan** of action	☐ Actively listened and validated expectations ☐ Showed empathy and used appropriate reassurances ☐ Inquired about patient's support system ☐ Managed the **challenge** (here; mother asked, "Will my baby be okay?")	

Viral gastroenteritis
Rotavirus
C dif

History and Physical Examination Checklist

HPI

- ☐ Vomiting
    - ☐ 6 episodes
    - ☐ Non bloody
    - ☐ Initially food particles only
    - ☐ Currently bilious
- ☐ Diarrhea
    - ☐ 4 episodes in the past day
    - ☐ Brown stools
    - ☐ Watery
    - ☐ Non bloody
    - ☐ Appears to be in pain with every bowel movement
- ☐ Duration: 2 days
- ☐ Onset
    - ☐ Sudden
    - ☐ 1 day after playdate
    - ☐ No known sick contacts
- ☐ Anorexia
    - ☐ Nothing PO
- ☐ Fever
    - ☐ Low grade fever
    - ☐ Improved with Tylenol
- ☐ No cough
- ☐ No rhinorrhea
- ☐ No shortness of breath
- ☐ No skin rashes or discoloration of the skin.

PMH

- ☐ Recent otitis media
    - ☐ Treated with amoxicillin
    - ☐ 4 weeks ago
- ☐ No hospitalizations
- ☐ No surgery
- ☐ No recent trauma
- ☐ Meds: Tylenol
- ☐ No other medications
- ☐ NKDA

Ped Hx

- ☐ Full term
- ☐ Delivered by elective cesarean section
- ☐ Adequate prenatal care
- ☐ Mother did not smoke, use drugs or alcohol during pregnancy
- ☐ Breastfed
    - ☐ 8 mos
- ☐ Currently eats
    - ☐ Regular table food
    - ☐ Drinks cow's milk
- ☐ Regular well child visits
    - ☐ Met age appropriate developmental milestones
- ☐ Immunization
    - ☐ Up to date
    - ☐ Except rotavirus

Family Hx

- ☐ Father and mother have no history of acute diarrhea
- ☐ No sick contacts

Social Hx

- ☐ Lives with parents
- ☐ Pet dog

Physical Examination

No physical exam

[handwritten: Stool culture in Rotavirus PCR]

Patient Note

History

HPI: 18 m/o girl with vomiting and diarrhea for past 3 days, started 1 day after playdate with other toddlers. Vomited 6 times, initially mostly food particles, now mostly bilious, but non-bloody. She has decreased appetite and poor PO intake. Stool is mostly watery and brown, without evidence of blood. She shows signs of cramps and abdominal pain with each BM. Has had a low-grade fever which improved with Tylenol. No skin rashes, no sick contacts.

PMHx: Otitis media treated with oral antibiotics 4 wks ago. No prior hospitalizations, surgeries, or trauma. Breastfed until 8 mos and now eats regular table food and cow's milk. Met age-appropriate developmental milestones. Immunizations up to date, except rotavirus vaccine.

Medications: Pediatric multivitamin, Tylenol PRN fever

Allergies: NKDA

FH: Mother and father are healthy with no chronic illnesses.

Physical Examination

N/A

DIAGNOSIS 1. VIRAL GASTROENTERITIS

History Findings	Physical Exam Findings
Low grade fever	N/A
Non bloody vomitus	
Non-bloody diarrhea	
Acute onset of symptoms	
Incomplete rotavirus vaccinations	
Abdominal pain	

DIAGNOSIS 2. CLOSTRIDIUM DIFFICILE COLITIS

History Findings	Physical Exam Findings
Low-grade fever	N/A
Diarrhea	
Recent antibiotic use	
Abdominal pain	

Diagnostic Studies

Physical exam

CBC w/ differential

Electrolytes, BUN, creatinine

Stool for *C. difficile* toxin / ELISA for toxin A or B / stool PCR for rotavirus

Stool for fecal leukocytes, ova and parasites

CASE 22: LACK OF ENERGY

Doorway Information

Opening Scenario

Mr. Dennis Hall is a 55-year-old man who presents with decreased energy for the past 3 yrs.

Vital Signs

T 98.0 F (36.6 C)

BP 130/85 mm Hg

Pulse 90/min

Respirations 12/min

Weight 250 lbs

Height 5 ft. 7 in.

Examinee Tasks

1. Obtain a focused history.

2. Perform a relevant physical exam. Do not perform rectal, pelvic, genitourinary, or corneal reflex exam.

3. Discuss your initial diagnostic impression and your workup plan with the patient.

4. After leaving the room, complete your Patient Note on the given form.

Communication and Interpersonal Skills Checklist

Fostering the Relationship	Gathering Information	Providing Information
☐ Knocked	☐ Elicited chief complaint	☐ Summarized significant information
☐ Introduced self	☐ Established timeline of patient's CC (chief complaint)	☐ Provided diagnostic impression
☐ Clarified role	☐ Used open-ended question	☐ Justified diagnosis with evidence from encounter
☐ Was properly groomed	☐ Used non-leading questions	☐ Assessed patient's need for additional information
☐ Made eye contact	☐ Used closed-ended questions	☐ Encouraged and answered questions
☐ Maintained appropriate distance	☐ Asked one question at a time	☐ Assessed patient's comprehension of probable illness
☐ Displayed confident manner	☐ Did not use medical jargon	
☐ Showed care and concern	☐ Appropriately used "continuers"	
☐ Was respectful and nonjudgmental	☐ Paraphrased	
☐ Established patient's preferred title	☐ Appropriately used transitions	
☐ Used proper draping	☐ Elicited additional concerns	
☐ Focused on patient	☐ Assessed impact on patient's life	
☐ Did not interrupt patient	☐ Checked for patient understanding	
☐ Maintained appropriate and responsive body language		

Making Decisions	Supporting Emotions
☐ Clearly stated next steps in management	☐ Actively listened and validated patient's expectations
☐ **Counseled** patient	☐ Showed empathy and used appropriate reassurances
☐ Agreed to **mutual plan** of action	☐ Inquired about patient's support system
	☐ Managed the **challenge** (here; patient asked, "is it normal to be forgetful at my age?")

History and Physical Examination Checklist

HPI

- ☐ Decreased energy
  - ☐ Duration: 3 yrs
  - ☐ Progressive
- ☐ Sleeps 8 hours
  - ☐ Does not snore (according to wife)
  - ☐ Does not need to take naps during the day
- ☐ Weight gain
  - ☐ 5 lbs
  - ☐ Over 1 year
  - ☐ Does not exercise
    - ☐ No energy
  - ☐ Tries to eat healthy
- ☐ Forgetfulness
  - ☐ Difficulty remembering clients' names
  - ☐ Forgets to complete tasks on time
  - ☐ Assumes it is due to age
- ☐ Numbness and tingling
  - ☐ Right hand
  - ☐ Occasional
  - ☐ Especially when he wakes up
- ☐ Strange feeling in legs
- ☐ Change in voice timber
  - ☐ Recent onset
  - ☐ Insidious
  - ☐ Hoarser voice
- ☐ Mild cold intolerance/no heat intolerance
- ☐ Constipation
  - ☐ Occasionally
- ☐ No diarrhea
- ☐ No chest pain
- ☐ No palpitations
- ☐ No SOB

(handwritten: depression / dementia)

(handwritten: laryngeal Cancer)

PMH

- ☐ No significant past medical history
- ☐ No hospitalization or surgery
- ☐ Meds: no prescription meds, Colace for constipation
- ☐ NKDA
- ☐ Has not seen a physician in 2 yrs

Family Hx

- ☐ Maternal uncle with Sjogren's syndrome
- ☐ No other significant family history

Social Hx

- ☐ Works as an accountant
- ☐ No recreational drugs
- ☐ No smoking
- ☐ No alcohol
- ☐ Married
- ☐ Monogamous with wife

Physical Examination

- ☐ Washed hands prior to examination
- ☐ Inspected hair
- ☐ Inspected skin
- ☐ Inspected thyroid gland
- ☐ Auscultated neck for thyroid bruits
- ☐ Palpated thyroid gland
- ☐ Palpated neck for all lymph nodes

- ☐ Performed mini mental status exam
- ☐ Assessed motor strength bilaterally in hands
- ☐ Assessed DTRs
- ☐ Assessed 2 modalities of sensation (light, sharp/dull) bilaterally
- ☐ Performed gait exam

Patient Note

History

HPI: 55 y/o man presents with decreasing energy for the past 3 yrs. He reports a 5-lb weight gain over the past 2 yrs. He also complains of moderate cold intolerance. He has not seen a physician in over 2 yrs. He works as an accountant and mentions being more forgetful lately. He also reports occasional numbness and tingling of his right hand. He denies thinning of his hair, changes in his diet, swelling of his legs. His wife reports that he does not snore at night but that his voice has become hoarser.

ROS: no chest pain, no SOB, occasional constipation, no diarrhea.

PMH/SHx: no hospitalizations, no previous surgeries

Meds: Colace, as needed for constipation, no herbal medications, no prescription meds.

Allergies: NKDA

Family Hx: Maternal uncle with Sjogren's syndrome

Social Hx: Pt is married, 3 children, monogamous with wife. No h/o EtoH, Smoking or Rec Drugs

Physical Exam

T 98.0 F; BP 130/85 mm Hg; pulse 90/min; respirations12/min

Gen: No acute distress. Overweight. Voice sounds hoarse

A&O x3

Neck: No carotid or thyroid bruit; No visible scars or swelling; No thyroid tenderness or enlargement

Neuro: motor strength: 5/5 UE b/I; DTR: 2+; light, dull sensations intact; sharp sensation decreased on palm, & front of thumb, index & middle finger of right hand;

Gait: normal

Skin: forearms dry & scaly

Data Interpretation

DIAGNOSIS 1. HYPOTHYROIDISM

History Findings	Physical Exam Findings
Fatigue	Overweight
Weight gain	Decreased sensation in right hand
Numbness in right hand	Skin dry and scaly
Constipation	
Voice change	
Cold intolerance	
Uncle with history of Sjogren's syndrome	
Impaired memory	

DIAGNOSIS 2. IRON DEFICIENCY ANEMIA

History Findings	Physical Exam Findings
Fatigue	Skin dry and scaly
Constipation	
Cold intolerance	
Leg cramps	

Diagnostic Studies

Rectal exam, FOB

TSH, T4, FTI

CBC, peripheral smear

Serum Fe, TIBC, serum ferritin

CASE 23: CHEST PAIN

Doorway Information

Opening Scenario

Mrs. Simone David, a 53-year-old woman, presents with chest pain for the past 2 hours.

Vital Signs

T 98.6 F (37 C);

BP 150/90 mm Hg

Pulse 86/min

Respirations 20/min

O2 97% on room air

Examinee Tasks

1. Obtain a focused history.

2. Perform a relevant physical exam. Do not perform rectal, pelvic, genitourinary, female breast, or corneal reflex exam.

3. Discuss your initial diagnostic impression and your workup plan with the patient.

4. After leaving the room, complete your Patient Note on the given form.

Communication and Interpersonal Skills Checklist

Fostering the Relationship	Gathering Information	Providing Information
☐ Knocked	☐ Elicited chief complaint	☐ Summarized significant information
☐ Introduced self	☐ Established timeline of patient's CC (chief complaint)	☐ Provided diagnostic impression
☐ Clarified role	☐ Used open-ended question	☐ Justified diagnosis with evidence from encounter
☐ Was properly groomed	☐ Used non-leading questions	☐ Assessed patient's need for additional information
☐ Made eye contact	☐ Used closed-ended questions	☐ Encouraged and answered questions
☐ Maintained appropriate distance	☐ Asked one question at a time	☐ Assessed patient's comprehension of probable illness
☐ Displayed confident manner	☐ Did not use medical jargon	
☐ Showed care and concern	☐ Appropriately used "continuers"	
☐ Was respectful and nonjudgmental	☐ Paraphrased	
☐ Established patient's preferred title	☐ Appropriately used transitions	
☐ Used proper draping	☐ Elicited additional concerns	
☐ Focused on patient	☐ Assessed impact on patient's life	
☐ Did not interrupt patient	☐ Checked for patient understanding	
☐ Maintained appropriate and responsive body language		

Making Decisions	Supporting Emotions
☐ Clearly stated next steps in management	☐ Actively listened and validated patient's expectations
☐ **Counseled** patient	☐ Showed empathy and used appropriate reassurances
☐ Agreed to **mutual plan** of action	☐ Inquired about patient's support system
	☐ Managed the **challenge** (here; patient asked, "Should I be worried?")

History and Physical Examination Checklist

HPI
- ☐ Chest pain
- ☐ Duration: 2 hours
- ☐ Acute onset
- ☐ Constant
- ☐ Sharp
- ☐ Not radiating
- ☐ 5/10 severity
- ☐ No change in pain with
  - ☐ Exercise
  - ☐ Feeding
  - ☐ Position
  - ☐ Deep inspiration
- ☐ No shortness of breath
- ☐ No palpitations
- ☐ No diaphoresis
- ☐ No recent travel
- ☐ No trauma
- ☐ No strenuous activity
  - ☐ Sport
  - ☐ Lifting heavy objects
- ☐ OBGYN
  - ☐ LMP
    - ☐ 2 weeks ago
    - ☐ Regular
  - ☐ Para 1
  - ☐ Gravida 1

aortic dissection

PMH
- ☐ No similar episodes in the past
- ☐ No recent injuries
- ☐ No history of HTN, heart disease, high cholesterol or diabetes
- ☐ No hospitalization or surgery except child birth
- ☐ LMP 2 wks ago
- ☐ No meds
- ☐ NKDA

Family Hx
- ☐ No family history of diabetes, heart disease, high cholesterol or hypertension

Social Hx
- ☐ No recreational drugs
- ☐ No Smoking
- ☐ Alcohol
  - ☐ 2 glasses of wine/week
- ☐ Married
- ☐ Monogamous
- ☐ No history of STDs

Physical Examination

- ☐ Washed hands prior to examination
- ☐ Inspection of chest & JVP
- ☐ Auscultation of 4 valves of heart and carotids
- ☐ Palpation of chest for tenderness, location of PMI,   *costochondritis*
  - ☐ Reproducible tenderness of the sternocostal angle
- ☐ Auscultation of lungs
- ☐ Checked carotid & peripheral pulses
- ☐ Examination of extremities for edema, clubbing and cyanosis

Patient Note

History

HPI: 53 y/o woman with no significant past medical history presents with acute onset of sharp, constant, non-radiating chest pain which began 2 hrs ago. Pain is 5/10 in severity, is not associated with shortness of breath or palpitations, and is non-pleuritic. The pain is not precipitated by food or exercise. She has no personal or family history of diabetes or heart disease. She takes no medications and denies recent travel history or heavy lifting.

PMH/PSHx: no hospitalization, no trauma, no past medical history

Meds: none

Allergies: NKDA

FHx: no contributory family history, no similar CC or illnesses

SxHx: married with 1 child. No history of sexually transmitted disease and is monogamous with her husband. (−) tobacco/illicit drug use, (+) EtOH 2 glasses of wine/wk.

Physical Examination

T 98.6 F; BP 150/90 mm Hg; pulse 86/min; respirations 20/min O2 97% RA

GA: alert, conscious and coherent; in moderate distress

CV: S1 and S2 normal; regular rate and rhythm; no murmurs, rubs or gallops; PMI not displaced; no carotid bruits; no JVD; positive point tenderness on sternocostal angle

Lung: clear to auscultation and percussion Bilaterally; no rales, wheezes, rhonchi or rubs; no bruises, swelling

Extremities: peripheral pulses palpable and equal Bilaterally, 2+; no clubbing, cyanosis or pedal edema

---

Data Interpretation

DIAGNOSIS 1: COSTOCHONDRITIS

History Findings	Physical Exam Findings
Chest pain	Normal pulse and O2 saturation
Acute onset	Point tenderness on sternocostal angle
Constant, non-radiating sharp pain	No palpable edema
Pain is non-pleuritic	
Not associated with SOB or palpitations	
No family h/o DM or heart disease	
No risk factors for heart disease	
No h/o HTN, DM, heart Dx	
No h/o cocaine use	

DIAGNOSIS 2: ACUTE MYOCARDIAL INFARCTION

History Findings	Physical Exam Findings
Chest pain: sharp, constant	Hypertensive: 150/90 mm Hg
Pain not precipitated by food or deep inspiration	
Acute onset	

Diagnostic Studies

EKG

Chest x-ray

CBC with diff, electrolytes, BUN/creatinine

CK-MB, troponin

CASE 24: KNEE AND GREAT TOE PAIN

Doorway Information

Opening Scenario

Mr. James Hopper is a 58-year-old man who presents with severe pain in his left knee and left great toe for the past 2 days.

Vital Signs

T 99.8 F (37.6 C)

BP 130/80 mm Hg

Pulse 88/min

Respirations 16/min

Examinee Tasks

1. Obtain a focused history.

2. Perform a relevant physical exam. Do not perform rectal, pelvic, genitourinary, female breast, or corneal reflex exam.

3. Discuss your initial diagnostic impression and your workup plan with the patient.

4. After leaving the room, complete your Patient Note on the given form.

Communication and Interpersonal Skills Checklist

Fostering the Relationship	Gathering Information	Providing Information
☐ Knocked	☐ Elicited chief complaint	☐ Summarized significant information
☐ Introduced self	☐ Established timeline of patient's CC (chief complaint)	☐ Provided diagnostic impression
☐ Clarified role	☐ Used open-ended question	☐ Justified diagnosis with evidence from encounter
☐ Was properly groomed	☐ Used non-leading questions	☐ Assessed patient's need for additional information
☐ Made eye contact	☐ Used closed-ended questions	☐ Encouraged and answered questions
☐ Maintained appropriate distance	☐ Asked one question at a time	☐ Assessed patient's comprehension of probable illness
☐ Displayed confident manner	☐ Did not use medical jargon	
☐ Showed care and concern	☐ Appropriately used "continuers"	
☐ Was respectful and nonjudgmental	☐ Paraphrased	
☐ Established patient's preferred title	☐ Appropriately used transitions	
☐ Used proper draping	☐ Elicited additional concerns	
☐ Focused on patient	☐ Assessed impact on patient's life	
☐ Did not interrupt patient	☐ Checked for patient understanding	
☐ Maintained appropriate and responsive body language		

Making Decisions	Supporting Emotions
☐ Clearly stated next steps in management	☐ Actively listened and validated patient's expectations
☐ **Counseled** patient	☐ Showed empathy and used appropriate reassurances
☐ Agreed to **mutual plan** of action	☐ Inquired about patient's support system
	☐ Managed the **challenge** (here; patient asked, "Can you give me something for the pain?")

History and Physical Examination Checklist

HPI
- ☐ Left knee pain
- ☐ Left great toe pain
- ☐ Burning sensation
- ☐ Acute onset
  - ☐ Woke him up from sleep
  - ☐ 2 night ago
- ☐ Intensity 9/10
- ☐ Feels sharp
  - ☐ Occasionally dull as well
- ☐ Does not radiate anywhere
- ☐ Increased warmth
- ☐ Swelling of knee and toe
- ☐ No history of trauma
- ☐ Alleviated by ibuprofen
  - ☐ 400 mg
  - ☐ Swelling subsided
  - ☐ Intensity 5/10
- ☐ Exacerbated by pressure from clothing and shoes
- ☐ Previous episode
  - ☐ 4 yrs ago
  - ☐ Also alleviated with ibuprofen
- ☐ No recent injuries to his foot or his knee
- ☐ Started swimming 2-3 per week to lose weight
- ☐ High protein diet
  - ☐ Red meat most days of the week

PMH
- ☐ Similar episode in past
- ☐ No x-ray taken at the time
- ☐ Did not seek medical attention
- ☐ No history of any chronic condition
- ☐ Meds
- ☐ No prescription meds
- ☐ OTC ibuprofen for past 2 days
- ☐ NKDA

Family Hx
- ☐ Non contributory

Social Hx
- ☐ Former smoker
- ☐ 1 pack/day
- ☐ Quit 10 yrs ago
- ☐ No recreational drugs
- ☐ No Alcohol
- ☐ Married
- ☐ Works as a photographer
- ☐ Is physically active

Physical Examination

- ☐ Washed hands prior to examination
- ☐ Inspection of upper and lower extremities
- ☐ Palpation of joints in upper and lower extremities
- ☐ Erythematous and tender to palpation
- ☐ Palpation of peripheral pulses
- ☐ Motor strength of upper and lower extremities
- ☐ Range of motion of upper, then lower, extremities
- ☐ Limited painful flexion and extension of affected joints

Patient Note

History

HPI: 58 y/o man with no significant past medical history presents with burning pain of the left knee and left big toe, which started 2 days ago. Pain is 9/10 in severity, non-radiating and is exacerbated by any pressure from clothing and shoes. He took ibuprofen, which improved the pain and swelling to 5/10 in intensity. He is also experiencing swelling and warmth of the left knee and hallux. He had similar pain 4 yrs ago for which he took ibuprofen and also improved his pain. At that time, he did not see his PMD and the pain went away within a few days. He denies recent trauma to his left knee and left toe. He does not drink alcohol but does eat red meat most days of the week.

PMH/PSHx: obesity, no major surgeries.

Meds: ibuprofen 1-2 tabs daily for past 2 days

FHx: noncontributory

SH: former smoker, quit 10 yrs ago. No EtOH or recreational drugs. Swims for exercise several times a week

Physical Exam

T 99.8 F; BP 130/80 mm Hg; pulse 88/min; respirations 16/min

General: Obese, in moderate distress due to pain of both left great toe and left knee

Extremities: peripheral pulses palpable and equal Bilaterally, 2+; no lesions, scars, bruises, discoloration or edema on upper and lower extremities

Musculoskeletal: erythematous swelling, warmth, and tenderness with limited and painful flexion and extension of the left knee and left hallux. Other joints of upper and lower extremities bilaterally are nontender and ROM WNL, motor strength 5/5 UE/LE.

Data Interpretation

DIAGNOSIS 1: ACUTE GOUT

History Findings	Physical Exam Findings
Pain in left patellar area and hallux with swelling and warmth	Tender, erythematous, with limited and painful flexion and extension of the left patella and left hallux
Pressure of shoe and clothing exacerbates pain	Swelling and warmth
No h/o trauma	Obesity
Pain improved with ibuprofen	
High protein diet (red meat)	
Acute onset	
Previous episode of resolved inflammatory arthritis	
No FH of autoimmune disease	

DIAGNOSIS 2. CALCIUM PYROPHOSPHATE DEPOSITION (PSEUDOGOUT)

History Findings	Physical Exam Findings
Pain in left patellar area and hallux with swelling and warmth	Tender, erythematous, with limited and painful flexion and extension of the left patella and left hallux
Pressure of shoe and clothing exacerbates pain	Swelling and warmth
No h/o trauma	
Pain improved with ibuoprofen	
Acute onset	
Previous episode of resolved inflammatory arthritis	

Diagnostic Studies

CBC with differential count

ESR, CRP, serum uric acid

Synovial fluid aspiration, fluid analysis with polarizing microscopy, cell count, C&S, Gram stain

X-ray of left knee and left hallux

[handwritten: Fluid analysis w/ polarizing microscopy c/s, gram stain]

CASE 25: SEVERE CHEST PAIN

Doorway Information

Opening Scenario

Mr. Dwyane Jackson is a 58-year-old man who presents with chest pain for past 1 hour.

Vital Signs

T 98.6 F (37 C)

BP 128/80 mm Hg

Pulse 110/min

Respirations 22/min

Examinee Tasks

1. Obtain a focused history.

2. Perform a relevant physical exam. Do not perform rectal, pelvic, genitourinary, female breast, or corneal reflex exam.

3. Discuss your initial diagnostic impression and your workup plan with the patient.

4. After leaving the room, complete your Patient Note on the given form.

Communication and Interpersonal Skills Checklist

Fostering the Relationship	Gathering Information	Providing Information
☐ Knocked	☐ Elicited chief complaint	☐ Summarized significant information
☐ Introduced self	☐ Established timeline of patient's CC (chief complaint)	☐ Provided diagnostic impression
☐ Clarified role	☐ Used open-ended question	☐ Justified diagnosis with evidence from encounter
☐ Was properly groomed	☐ Used non-leading questions	☐ Assessed patient's need for additional information
☐ Made eye contact	☐ Used closed-ended questions	☐ Encouraged and answered questions
☐ Maintained appropriate distance	☐ Asked one question at a time	☐ Assessed patient's comprehension of probable illness
☐ Displayed confident manner	☐ Did not use medical jargon	
☐ Showed care and concern	☐ Appropriately used "continuers"	
☐ Was respectful and nonjudgmental	☐ Paraphrased	
☐ Established patient's preferred title	☐ Appropriately used transitions	
☐ Used proper draping	☐ Elicited additional concerns	
☐ Focused on patient	☐ Assessed impact on patient's life	
☐ Did not interrupt patient	☐ Checked for patient understanding	
☐ Maintained appropriate and responsive body language		

Making Decisions	Supporting Emotions
☐ Clearly stated next steps in management	☐ Actively listened and validated patient's expectations
☐ **Counseled** patient	☐ Showed empathy and used appropriate reassurances
☐ Agreed to **mutual plan** of action	☐ Inquired about patient's support system
	☐ Managed the **challenge** (here; patient asked, "Am I having a heart attack?")

Panic attack
ACS
esophageal spasm

History and Physical Examination Checklist

HPI

- ☐ Chest pain
  - ☐ Substernal
  - ☐ 7/10 intensity
  - ☐ No radiation
- ☐ Duration 1 hour
- ☐ Started while moving furniture into son's new apartment
- ☐ Prior to pain, patient had a meal at a diner
- ☐ Patient stressed because son is relocating to attend college
- ☐ Pain not relieved by rest
- ☐ SOB
- ☐ No diaphoresis
- ☐ No nausea
- ☐ No recent weight loss or gain
- ☐ Eats a healthy diet

PMH

- ☐ No similar episodes in the past
- ☐ No hospitalizations or surgeries
- ☐ Meds
- ☐ No prescription meds
- ☐ Daily multivitamin
- ☐ NKDA

Family Hx

- ☐ Father deceased from "heart trouble"
- ☐ Age 67
- ☐ Mother with history of DM and HTN

Social Hx

- ☐ Retired police officer
- ☐ No alcohol
- ☐ No recreational drugs
- ☐ No smoking

Physical Examination

- ☐ Washed hands prior to examination
- ☐ Auscultated the carotids
- ☐ Palpated peripheral pulses bilaterally (radial, DP, PT pulse)
- ☐ Inspected thorax
- ☐ Examined for JVD
- ☐ Palpated chest wall
- ☐ Palpated PMI
- ☐ Auscultated heart in 4 areas
- ☐ Auscultated lungs
- ☐ Inspected abdomen
- ☐ Auscultated abdomen
- ☐ Palpated abdomen in 4 quadrants
- ☐ Examined for clubbing, cyanosis, and edema

Patient Note

History

HPI: 58 y/o man presents with sharp (7/10) sub-sternal chest pain without radiation for 1 hour duration. Started while moving furniture. He and his son had just eaten at a local diner. He is under a lot of stress due to his son relocating for college. SOB but no diaphoresis or nausea. There are no prior episodes of chest pain. He did not take anything for this pain and tried resting, which did not help his symptoms.

PMH/PSHx: no chronic medical history, no previous surgeries

Meds: multivitamins

Allergies: NKDA

FH: Father deceased at age 67 of "heart trouble," mother alive with HTN, DM2

SH: Retired police officer, nonsmoker, no h/o EtOH, no recreational drugs

Physical Exam

T 98.6 F; BP 128/80 mm Hg; pulse 110/min; respirations 22/min

General: patient appears anxious and in severe distress, holding his chest

Neck: no carotid bruits, no JVD

Cardiac: S1 S2 tachycardic, no M/G/R, no chest wall tenderness, PMI not displaced

Lungs: CTA bilaterally

Abd: soft, NT/ND, no hepatosplenomegaly, no rebound, no guarding, bowel sounds present

Extremities: peripheral pulses +2 and equal bilaterally, no lesions, scars, bruises, discoloration or edema on upper and lower extremities

Data Interpretation

DIAGNOSIS 1. ACUTE MYOCARDIAL INFARCTION

History Findings	Physical Exam Findings
Age >55	Tachycardia
Gender male	Tachypnea
Severe chest pain following strenuous activity	Pt appears to be in severe distress
Substernal location	Cardiac examination without chest wall tenderness
1 hour duration	
Associated SOB	
Not relieved by rest	
Family history of "heart trouble," DM2, and HTN	

DIAGNOSIS 2. ANGINA PECTORIS

History Findings	Physical Exam Findings
Age and gender	Tachycardia
Chest pain following strenuous activity	No tenderness to palpation on examination of chest
Sharp substernal chest pain	Pt in severe distress
Associated SOB	
FH of heart Dx	

DIAGNOSIS 3. ESOPHAGEAL SPASM

History Findings	Physical Exam Findings
Chest pain after eating meal	Normal BP
Stress due to son's relocation	
Not relieved by rest	
No prior episodes of chest pain with exercise	
Severe retrosternal pain	
1 hour duration	

Diagnostic Studies

CBC w/ differential

Serum electrolytes, BUN/creatinine, glucose

Troponin, CK-MB

EKG

CXR

Echocardiogram

CASE 26: CONFUSION, BLURRY VISION, AND SHORTNESS OF BREATH

Doorway Information

Opening Scenario

Ms. Robin Harrison is a 48-year-old woman who presents with confusion, blurry vision, and shortness of breath for the past 3 hours.

Vital Signs

T 98.6 F (37 C)

BP 230/130 mm Hg   — HTN emergency

Pulse 88/min

Respirations 22/min

O2 saturation 98% on room air

Examinee Tasks

1. Obtain a focused history.

2. Perform a relevant physical exam. Do not perform rectal, pelvic, genitourinary, female breast, or corneal reflex exam.

3. Discuss your initial diagnostic impression and your workup plan with the patient.

4. After leaving the room, complete your Patient Note on the given form.

Communication and Interpersonal Skills Checklist

Fostering the Relationship	Gathering Information	Providing Information
☐ Knocked ☐ Introduced self ☐ Clarified role ☐ Was properly groomed ☐ Made eye contact ☐ Maintained appropriate distance ☐ Displayed confident manner ☐ Showed care and concern ☐ Was respectful and nonjudgmental ☐ Established patient's preferred title ☐ Used proper draping ☐ Focused on patient ☐ Did not interrupt patient ☐ Maintained appropriate and responsive body language	☐ Elicited chief complaint ☐ Established timeline of patient's CC (chief complaint) ☐ Used open-ended question ☐ Used non-leading questions ☐ Used closed-ended questions ☐ Asked one question at a time ☐ Did not use medical jargon ☐ Appropriately used "continuers" ☐ Paraphrased ☐ Appropriately used transitions ☐ Elicited additional concerns ☐ Assessed impact on patient's life ☐ Checked for patient understanding	☐ Summarized significant information ☐ Provided diagnostic impression ☐ Justified diagnosis with evidence from encounter ☐ Assessed patient's need for additional information ☐ Encouraged and answered questions ☐ Assessed patient's comprehension of probable illness

Making Decisions	Supporting Emotions
☐ Clearly stated next steps in management ☐ **Counseled** patient ☐ Agreed to **mutual plan** of action	☐ Actively listened and validated patient's expectations ☐ Showed empathy and used appropriate reassurances ☐ Inquired about patient's support system ☐ Managed the **challenge** (here; patient asked, "Am I having a heart attack?")

History and Physical Examination Checklist

HPI

☐ Confusion
☐ Blurry vision
☐ Shortness of breath
☐ Duration 3 hour
☐ Symptoms worse over past hour
☐ Started while she was seated at her desk
☐ Presenting symptoms
    ☐ Headache
    ☐ Dizziness
    ☐ Palpitations
☐ No fever
☐ No chills
☐ No Nausea
☐ No vomiting

PMH

☐ No similar episodes in the past
☐ HTN, migraine headaches
☐ Meds: hydrochlorothiazide
☐ No hospitalizations or surgery, except for childbirths
☐ NKDA
☐ OBGYN
    ☐ LMP 2 weeks ago
    ☐ G2P2
    ☐ No miscarriages
    ☐ No contraceptive pills

Family Hx

☐ No family history of hypertension, diabetes or heart disease

Social Hx

☐ Alcohol
☐ 1-2 glasses of wine/month
☐ No recreational drugs
☐ No smoking
☐ Works as a secretary

Physical Examination

☐ Washed hands prior to examination
☐ Examined cranial nerves II–XII
☐ Performed fundoscopic examination
☐ Assessed mental status
☐ Examined motor strength
☐ Examined sensation
☐ Examined deep tendon reflexes
☐ Examined cerebellar function
☐ Examined gait and tested for Romberg sign
☐ Examined for JVD
☐ Auscultated heart
☐ Auscultated lungs
☐ Palpated peripheral pulses
☐ Examined extremities for edema/clubbing/cyanosis

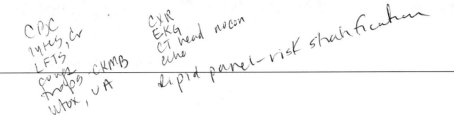

Patient Note

History

HPI: 48 y/o woman presents with confusion, blurry vision, and shortness of breath for 3 hours. She works as a secretary and was sitting at her desk when she suddenly developed these symptoms. She also complains of headache, dizziness, and palpitations. She denies having fever, chills, nausea, or vomiting. The only symptom she has had previously is headache. She takes hydrochlorothiazide for long-standing HTN, and does not use tobacco products or illicit drugs. She drinks 1-2 glasses of wine a month. Her LMP was 2 weeks ago.

ROS: no chest pain, no abd pain, no diarrhea/constipation/nausea/vomiting

PMH/PSHx: HTN, migraine headaches, no previous surgeries

Meds: hydrochlorothiazide. No over-the-counter medications

Allergies: NKDA

Family history: no HTN, DM2, or heart disease

Physical Examination

VS: T 98.6 F; BP 230/150 mm Hg; pulse 88/min; respirations 16/min

General: Patient in moderate distress, dyspneic

HEENT: PERRLA, EOM intact, no visual field defects, no carotid bruits, no JVD

Fundoscopic exam: sharp disc margins (no papilledema), no hemorrhages or exudates, + AV nicking

CV: S1/S2 WNL, RRR, no m, r, or g

Respiratory: CTA bilaterally, no wheezes, crackles, or rhonchi

Extremities: +2 pulses, no cyanosis, clubbing or edema

Neuro: CN II–XII intact, UE and LE: DTR 2+ bilateral; sharp/dull sensation intact Bilaterally; muscle strength 5/5 Bilaterally, cerebellar function intact

Data Interpretation

Diagnosis 1. Hypertensive crisis

History Findings	Physical Exam Findings
H/O HTN	BP 230/150 mm Hg
Blurry vision	Patient in moderate distress
Confusion	Dyspnea
Associated headache	No focal neurological findings
Dizziness	
Palpitations	
Dyspnea	

DIAGNOSIS 2. CEREBROVASCULAR ACCIDENT

History Findings	Physical Exam Findings
Blurry vision	BP 230/150 mm Hg
Confusion	Patient in moderate distress
Associated headache	
Dizziness	
H/O HTN	

DIAGNOSIS 3. ANGINA DUE TO VASOSPASM

History Findings	Physical Exam Findings
Dyspnea	Patient in moderate distress
Palpitations	AV nicking (artherosclerosis evidence)
H/O HTN, migraines	

Diagnostic Studies

CBC w/ differential

Cholesterol, HDL, LDL, triglycerides

CK-MB, troponin

EKG

CT scan head

BUN/Cr

U/A - protein

Chest x-ray

CASE 27: LIFE INSURANCE REQUEST

Doorway Information

Opening Scenario

Mr. John Brown is a 55-year-old man who comes in today for a physical examination.

Vital Signs

Temp 37.0° C (98.6° F)

BP 145/94 mm Hg, right upper limb sitting

Pulse 90/min, regular

Respirations 20/min

Examinee Tasks

1. Obtain a focused history.

2. Perform a relevant physical exam. Do not perform rectal, pelvic, genitourinary, female breast, or corneal reflex exams.

3. Discuss your initial diagnostic impression and diagnostic plan with the patient.

4. After leaving the room, complete the standard patient form that is waiting for you at your desk.

5. Turn in the form that Mr. Brown gives you, but do not write on it.

Communication and Interpersonal Skills Checklist

Fostering the Relationship	Gathering Information	Providing Information
☐ Knocked ☐ Introduced self ☐ Clarified role ☐ Was properly groomed ☐ Made eye contact ☐ Maintained appropriate distance ☐ Displayed confident manner ☐ Showed care and concern ☐ Was respectful and nonjudgmental ☐ Established patient's preferred title ☐ Used proper draping ☐ Focused on patient ☐ Did not interrupt patient ☐ Maintained appropriate and responsive body language	☐ Elicited chief complaint ☐ Established timeline of patient's CC (chief complaint) ☐ Used open-ended question ☐ Used non-leading questions ☐ Used closed-ended questions ☐ Asked one question at a time ☐ Did not use medical jargon ☐ Appropriately used "continuers" ☐ Paraphrased ☐ Appropriately used transitions ☐ Elicited additional concerns ☐ Assessed impact on patient's life ☐ Checked for patient understanding	☐ Summarized significant information ☐ Provided diagnostic impression ☐ Justified diagnosis with evidence from encounter ☐ Assessed patient's need for additional information ☐ Encouraged and answered questions ☐ Assessed patient's comprehension of probable illness

Making Decisions	Supporting Emotions
☐ Clearly stated next steps in management ☐ **Counseled** patient ☐ Agreed to **mutual plan** of action	☐ Actively listened and validated patient's expectations ☐ Showed empathy and used appropriate reassurances ☐ Inquired about patient's support system ☐ Managed the **challenge** (here; patient asked, "This isn't a real physical, is it?")

History and Physical Examination Checklist

HPI

- [ ] No fever
- [ ] No chills
- [ ] No cough
- [ ] No SOB
- [ ] No Chest pain
- [ ] No changes in bowel habits
- [ ] No blood in the stool
- [ ] No unintentional weight loss
- [ ] Weight gain
  - [ ] 15 lbs
  - [ ] In 6 mos
  - [ ] Patient feels weight gain is due to sedentary job and eating habits
- [ ] Diet
  - [ ] High carbohydrate content
  - [ ] High fat content
  - [ ] Often feels hungry
- [ ] Increased urination
  - [ ] Increased frequency
  - [ ] Increased volume
  - [ ] No burning with urination
  - [ ] No blood in urine
  - [ ] No change in the urine stream
  - [ ] Nocturia
  - [ ] Challenging because of job
- [ ] Increased sleep
  - [ ] More than usual
  - [ ] Yet awakes tired
  - [ ] Wife relates that he snores
- [ ] Increased thirst
- [ ] No hoarseness of voice
- [ ] No trouble swallowing
- [ ] Erectile dysfunction

ROS

diet

PMH

- [ ] HTN
- [ ] Which patient believes is white coat syndrome
  - [ ] 10 yr history
- [ ] Meds: saw palmetto for increased frequency of urination
- [ ] Cholecystectomy 5 yrs ago
- [ ] NKDA

Family Hx

- [ ] Father and older brother deceased from heart attacks

Social Hx

- [ ] Alcohol
- [ ] 1-2 glasses of wine/week
- [ ] No recreational drugs
- [ ] Past history of smoking tobacco
  - [ ] 1 pack/day
  - [ ] 20 yrs
  - [ ] Quit 1 year ago
- [ ] Works as an air traffic controller
- [ ] Married with no children
- [ ] Not currently sexually active

Physical Examination

- [ ] Washed hands prior to examination
- [ ] Palpated lymph nodes
- [ ] Auscultated for carotid bruits
- [ ] Auscultated heart
- [ ] Palpated peripheral pulses
- [ ] Auscultated lungs
- [ ] Auscultated abdomen
- [ ] Palpated abdomen in 4 quadrants
- [ ] Examined DTRs
- [ ] Checked sensation in extremities
- [ ] Examined extremities for clubbing, cyanosis and edema

Patient Note

History

HPI: 55 y/o man comes in for an insurance physical. He has no present complaints and denies having any shortness of breath, chest pain, headache, blood in stool, cough, fever, nausea, vomiting, diarrhea, constipation, hoarseness of voice, or trouble swallowing. Increased somnolence and still wakes up tired. His wife mentioned that he snores loudly at night. He also reports a 15-lb weight gain over the past 6 mos. He has noticed that he has been urinating more frequently at night and during the daytime as well. He also notes increased thirst throughout the day and hunger even after a large meal. He denies dysuria and hematuria, disturbance in flow of urine, or hesitancy with urination.

PMH/SH: patient suspects HTN diagnosis is the "white coat syndrome"

Medications: saw palmetto for frequent urination

Allergies: NKDA

Family Hx: father and older brother both died due to MIs

Social Hx: married and lives with his wife. Smoked 1 PPD x 20 yrs, quit 1 year ago, drinks 1-2 glasses of wine per week. No illicit drug use. Works as an air traffic controller. Lives a rather sedentary life and eats a diet high in fat and carbohydrates. He is not currently sexually active with his wife as he has difficulty maintaining an erection.

Physical Exam

T 98.6 F, BP 145/94 mm Hg, right upper limb sitting, pulse 90/min, regular, pulse 20/min

GA: obese individual; not ill appearing

HEENT: no LAD, no carotid bruits

CV: +S1, S2, no m, r, g; RRR

Lungs: CTA bilaterally

Abdomen: cholecystectomy scar, 5 cm in RUQ, + BS in all 4 quadrants, soft, nontender, nondistended, no organomegaly

Ext: no cyanosis or clubbing, edema

Pulses: 2+ throughout

Neuro: diminished sensation in stocking pattern in lower extremities. Feet have no open sores or tenderness. DTRs: 2+ bilaterally

Data Interpretation

DIAGNOSIS 1. DIABETES TYPE II

History Findings	Physical Exam Findings
Weight gain	Obesity
Increased urinary frequency	Decreased sensation on neuro exam
Hyperphagia	Hypertension
Polydipsia	
Erectile dysfunction	

DIAGNOSIS 2. OBSTRUCTIVE SLEEP APNEA

History Findings	Physical Exam Findings
Daytime fatigue/tiredness	Obesity
Snoring at night, loud	Hypertension
Increased sleepiness during daytime	
Weight gain	
Nocturia	
Sexual dysfuction	
Male sex	

Diagnostic Studies

Fasting blood glucose
HgA1c
Polysomnography

° Constitutional
° HEENT
° Resp
° CV
° abd d/4l
° GU
° MSK
° HEME
° Neuro
° endo

ROS
- Vision hearing Δ epistaxis Δ
- SOB, cough, snoring
- CP, palpitations, orthopnea
- N/V, dysphagia, diar, constip, abd pain, bloody BM
- itching, skin Δ, jaundice
- polyuria, dypsia, heat/cold intol
- easy bruis, bleed
- Syncope, tremor, dizziness, HA, sensory Δ
- Swollen glands
- swollen joints

CASE 28: PRE-EMPLOYMENT PHYSICAL

Doorway Information

Opening Scenario

Mr. Robert Davis is a 40-year-old man who presents for a pre-employment physical examination.

Vital Signs

Temp 38.1°C (100.6°F)   *Febrile, tachy*

BP 140/90 mm Hg, right upper limb sitting

Pulse 110/min, regular

Respirations 20/min

Examinee Tasks

1. Obtain a focused history.

2. Perform a relevant physical exam. Do not perform rectal, pelvic, genitourinary, female breast, or corneal reflex exams.

3. Discuss your initial diagnostic impression and your workup plan with the patient.

4. After leaving the room, complete your Patient Note on the given form.

Communication and Interpersonal Skills Checklist		
Fostering the Relationship	**Gathering Information**	**Providing Information**
☐ Knocked ☐ Introduced self ☐ Clarified role ☐ Was properly groomed ☐ Made eye contact ☐ Maintained appropriate distance ☐ Displayed confident manner ☐ Showed care and concern ☐ Was respectful and nonjudgmental ☐ Established patient's preferred title ☐ Used proper draping ☐ Focused on patient ☐ Did not interrupt patient ☐ Maintained appropriate and responsive body language	☐ Elicited chief complaint ☐ Established timeline of patient's CC (chief complaint) ☐ Used open-ended question ☐ Used non-leading questions ☐ Used closed-ended questions ☐ Asked one question at a time ☐ Did not use medical jargon ☐ Appropriately used "continuers" ☐ Paraphrased ☐ Appropriately used transitions ☐ Elicited additional concerns ☐ Assessed impact on patient's life ☐ Checked for patient understanding	☐ Summarized significant information ☐ Provided diagnostic impression ☐ Justified diagnosis with evidence from encounter ☐ Assessed patient's need for additional information ☐ Encouraged and answered questions ☐ Assessed patient's comprehension of probable illness
Making Decisions	**Supporting Emotions**	
☐ Clearly stated next steps in management ☐ **Counseled** patient ☐ Agreed to **mutual plan** of action	☐ Actively listened and validated patient's expectations ☐ Showed empathy and used appropriate reassurances ☐ Inquired about patient's support system ☐ Managed the **challenge** (here; ask CAGE questions)	

History and Physical Examination Checklist

HPI

- ☐ No cough
- ☐ No SOB
- ☐ No chest pain
- ☐ No palpitations
- ☐ No dysuria
- ☐ No change in bowel habits
- ☑ 2 episodes of nausea and vomiting
- ☐ No abdominal pain
- ☐ No diarrhea
- ☐ No constipation
- ☐ No numbness/tingling
- ☐ No weight loss
- ☐ No night sweats
- ☐ No joint pain
- ☐ No bruises
- ☐ No difficulty with his hearing or eyesight
- ☑ Feels cold and clammy today
  - ☐ Sometimes feels this way
  - ☐ Goes away in a day or two
  - ☐ Thinks it's a virus
  - ☐ Feels fine otherwise
- ☐ No headache
- ☐ No blurry vision or changes in vision

EtOH use disorder
ETOH withdrawal

PMH

- ☐ No history of chronic illness
- ☐ No prior surgeries
- ☐ Hospitalization last month
- ☐ Concussion
- ☐ Required 4 stitches
- ☐ Can't remember what happened
- ☐ Urinated on clothing *?*
- ☐ NKDA
- ☐ No meds

Family Hx

- ☐ Family medical history unknown

Social Hx

- ☐ Not married
- ☐ Lives alone
- ☐ Currently between jobs
- ☐ Alcohol
  - ☐ 6 packs of beer on the weekend
  - ☐ Sometimes during the week as well
  - ☐ Drinks to stop the shakes
  - ☑ Has blackouts
  - ☐ CAGE (3 of 4)
- ☐ Uses recreational drugs
  - ☐ Marijuana
- ☐ Smoker
  - ☐ 1.5 packs/day
  - ☐ 20 yrs
- ☐ Works as a secretary

Physical Examination

- ☐ Washed hands prior to examination
- ☐ Inspected skin (spider angioma and palmar erythema)
  - ☐ diaphoretic and tremulous
  - ☐ spider angioma on the face
  - ☐ extremities show palmar erythema
- ☐ Inspected oropharynx
- ☐ Assessed mental status
  - ☐ His speech is somewhat slow
  - ☐ He does not make eye contact with you
  - ☐ Short-term memory is poor
  - ☐ He cannot repeat 3 words, nor can he spell the word world backward
  - ☐ He can name 3 objects
  - ☐ He does obey commands

liver failure
Wernicke Karsikof

- ☐ Examined cranial nerves II-XII
  - ☐ Extraocular movement appears intact but lateral nystagmus is seen
- ☐ Examined motor strength
  - ☐ Motor strength is normal on left arm and leg, though right arm and leg are noticeably weaker
- ☐ Examined sensation
- ☐ Examined DTRs
- ☐ Assessed cerebellar function
  - ☐ Gait is ataxic
- ☐ Auscultated heart and lungs
- ☐ Performed fundoscopic exam
- ☐ Abdominal exam

Patient Note

History

HPI: 40 y/o man requests pre-employment physical clearance. His speech is somewhat slow and slurred, and he presents with tremors, fever, and healing cuts on his forehead. He had 2 episodes of nausea and vomiting, no blood.

Patient reports that he frequently needs a drink in the morning to prevent "the shakes." He suspects he should feel guilty, and he sometimes wakes up on the floor with loss of urine and isn't sure what happened. He used to be very annoyed by his ex-wife criticizing his drinking, but she left last year.

Meds: none; NKDA

PMH: 1 hosp last month for head trauma, no surgery

SH: lives alone; smoking 30-pack yrs; occ marijuana, binge drinks >6 drinks at a time

CAGE (+) 3 out of 4; drinks frequently to stop shakes

?C AGE

Physical Exam

T 100.62 F, BP 140/90 mm Hg, pulse 110/min, respirations 20/min

GA: unkempt, dirty, and tremulous. Speech slow and slurred

Skin: palmar erythema, spider angioma

HEENT: healing, still-tender laceration to forehead. PERRLA, EOMI, + nystagmus

Fundoscopy: no papilledema

CV: S1 S2 WNL, RRR, no murmur, rub, and gallop, CTAB

Neuro: A + 0 X 2. Poor memory and concentration. Obeys commands and language is intact

Motor RUE and RLE 3/5. Left side 5/5. Sensation intact. Gait: ataxic; DTR 2+ throughout

Abd: bowel sounds present, nontender, no HSM

Data Interpretation

DIAGNOSIS 1. SUBDURAL HEMATOMA ✗ Chronic subdural

History Findings	Physical Exam Findings
History of concussion last month	A + O x 2, states year is 1995
Speech somewhat slow, slurred	Poor memory and concentration
"Woke up" on floor	Motor weakness on RUE and RLE 3/5
Incontinence	Laceration to head
2 episodes of nausea and vomiting	+ nystagmus
Risk factor: alcoholism	Gait: ataxic

DIAGNOSIS 2. WERNICKE ENCEPHALOPATHY

History Findings	Physical Exam Findings
Tremors	A + O x 2, states year is 1995
Speech somewhat slow, slurred	Poor memory and concentration
Incontinence	Motor weakness on RUE and RLE 3/5
Binge drinking >6 drinks at a time	Palmar erythema/spider angiomata
CAGE 3/4 positive	Nystagmus
2 episodes of nausea and vomiting	Gait: ataxic
	Tachycardia

DIAGNOSIS 3. ALCOHOL WITHDRAWAL SYNDROME

History Findings	Physical Exam Findings
Tremors	Palmar erythema/spider angiomata
Speech somewhat slow, slurred	A + O x 2, states year is 1995
History of concussion last month	Poor memory and concentration
Incontinence	Tachycardia
Woke up on floor	Fever
Binge drinking >6 drinks at a time	
CAGE 3/4 positive	
2 episodes of nausea and vomiting	

Diagnostic Studies

PT/PPT/INR, platelet count

CBC w/diff, glucose, ammonia level

Serum EtOH levels

CT/MRI of head

Total bilirubin, AST, ALT, GGT

EEG

Vit B1 level

CASE 29: MEDICATION REFILL

Doorway Information

Opening Scenario

Mr. Paul Thomas is a 49-year-old man who calls to request a refill of his medication.

Vital Signs

No vital signs are given in this case.

Examinee Tasks

1. Obtain a focused history.

2. Discuss your initial diagnostic impression and your workup plan with the patient.

3. After ending the call, complete your Patient Note on the given form.

Communication and Interpersonal Skills Checklist

Fostering the Relationship	Gathering Information	Providing Information
☐ Introduced self ☐ Clarified role ☐ Maintained appropriate distance ☐ Displayed confident manner ☐ Showed care and concern ☐ Was respectful and nonjudgmental ☐ Established preferred title ☐ Did not interrupt	☐ Elicited chief complaint ☐ Established timeline of patient's CC (chief complaint) ☐ Used open-ended question ☐ Used non-leading questions ☐ Used closed-ended questions ☐ Asked one question at a time ☐ Did not use medical jargon ☐ Appropriately used "continuers" ☐ Paraphrased ☐ Appropriately used transitions ☐ Elicited additional concerns ☐ Assessed impact on patient's life ☐ Checked for understanding	☐ Summarized significant information ☐ Provided diagnostic impression ☐ Justified diagnosis with evidence from encounter ☐ Assessed patient's need for additional information ☐ Encouraged and answered questions ☐ Assessed patient's comprehension of probable illness

Making Decisions	Supporting Emotions
☐ Clearly stated next steps in management ☐ **Counseled** patient ☐ Agreed to **mutual plan** of action	☐ Actively listened and validated patient's expectations ☐ Showed empathy and used appropriate reassurances ☐ Inquired about patient's support system ☐ Managed the **challenge** (here; patient asked, "are these questions really necessary?")

History and Physical Examination Checklist	
HPI C HF	**PMH**
☐ Checks BP regularly	☐ No hospitalization, no surgeries
☐ Systolic	☐ No history of diabetes, cancer, or heart disease
☐ 120-130 mmHg	☐ HTN
☐ Diastolic	☐ Medications: lisinopril 10 mg PO daily
☐ 70-84mmHg	☐ Compliant with medication
☐ No fever	☐ On drug for 4 yrs
☐ No headaches	☐ Last physician visit 14 mos ago
☐ No changes in vision	☐ NKDA
☐ No chest pain	**Family Hx**
☐ Mild SOB	☐ No family history of hypertension, diabetes or heart disease
☐ When climbing 2 flights of stairs	**Social Hx**
☐ Ankle edema	☐ Lives at home with wife of 25 yrs
☐ Dry cough	☐ Works as an accountant
☐ Symptoms in the past 2 mos	☐ No alcohol
☐ Weight gain	☐ No recreational drugs
☐ 15 lbs	☐ No smoking
☐ Over 2 mos	
☐ Recently needs more pillows to sleep	

Physical Examination
No physical exam

Patient Note

History

HPI: 49 y/o man calls to request a refill of his medication. He has a history of well-controlled hypertension for the past 10 yrs and is currently taking lisinopril 10 mg daily. He does report lower extremity edema, dry cough, and dyspnea on exertion for the past 2 mos. He has also gained 15 lbs over the past 6 mos. He also reports having to use 1 additional pillow to sleep at night over a similar timeframe. He denies fever/chills, change in appetite, headaches, changes in his vision, and chest pain. He works as an accountant and reports no changes in his level of stress. His last visit to the doctor was 14 months ago.

PMH/PSH: well-controlled hypertension. No prior surgeries.

Meds: lisinopril 10 mg PO daily

Allergies: NKDA

Family Hx: no HTN, diabetes, or heart disease

Social Hx: married, works as an accountant; denies EtOH, tobacco products, and drugs

Physical Exam

N/A

Data Interpretation

Diagnosis 1. Congestive heart failure

History Findings	Physical Exam Findings
History of HTN	N/A
15-lb weight gain	
Dyspnea on exertion	
2-pillow orthopnea	
LE edema	
Nonproductive cough	

Diagnosis 2. Renal insufficiency

History Findings	Physical Exam Findings
History of HTN	N/A
LE edema	
Dyspnea on exertion	
15-lb weight gain	
Use of lisinopril	

Diagnosis 3. Drug-induced cough

History Findings	Physical Exam Findings
Use of lisinopril	N/A
Non-productive cough	
No fever or chills	

Diagnostic Studies

Physical examination

CBC w/ diff

Serum electrolytes, BUN/creatinine, albumin, BNP

Total cholesterol, HDL, LDL, triglycerides

UA, urine electrolytes

EKG

Chest x-ray

Echocardiogram

CASE 30: BREAKING BAD NEWS

Doorway Information

Opening Scenario

Mr. Paul Harris is a 68-year-old man who had a prostate biopsy last week and is here to receive the pathology results. The results show he has adenocarcinoma of the prostate, and your task is to inform him.

Vital Signs

No vital signs are given in this case.

Examinee Tasks

1. Tell the patient he has prostate cancer.

2. There is no physical exam in this case.

3. Elicit original chief complaint and obtain HPI based on that complaint.

4. In the Patient Note, consider other diagnoses for that complaint.

Communication and Interpersonal Skills Checklist

Fostering the Relationship	Gathering Information	Providing Information
☐ Knocked	☐ Elicited chief complaint	☐ Summarized significant information
☐ Introduced self	☐ Established timeline of patient's CC (chief complaint)	☐ Provided diagnostic impression
☐ Clarified role	☐ Used open-ended question	☐ Justified diagnosis with evidence from encounter
☐ Was properly groomed	☐ Used non-leading questions	☐ Assessed patient's need for additional information
☐ Made eye contact	☐ Used closed-ended questions	☐ Encouraged and answered questions
☐ Maintained appropriate distance	☐ Asked one question at a time	☐ Assessed patient's comprehension of probable illness
☐ Displayed confident manner	☐ Did not use medical jargon	
☐ Showed care and concern	☐ Appropriately used "continuers"	
☐ Was respectful and nonjudgmental	☐ Paraphrased	
☐ Established patient's preferred title	☐ Appropriately used transitions	
☐ Used proper draping	☐ Elicited additional concerns	
☐ Focused on patient	☐ Assessed impact on patient's life	
☐ Did not interrupt patient	☐ Checked for patient understanding	
☐ Maintained appropriate and responsive body language		

Making Decisions	Supporting Emotions
☐ Clearly stated next steps in management	☐ Actively listened and validated patient's expectations
☐ **Counseled** patient	☐ Showed empathy and used appropriate reassurances
☐ Agreed to **mutual plan** of action	☐ Inquired about patient's support system
	☐ Managed the **challenge** (here; patient asked, "what are my options?")

History and Physical Examination Checklist	
HPI	**PMH**
☐ Positive results of recent prostate biopsy	☐ Hospitalized for tonsillectomy at age 13
☐ Difficulty urinating	☐ Meds: daily multivitamin
☐ Increased urgency	☐ NKDA
☐ Hesitancy initiating urination	**Family Hx**
☐ Weak urinary stream	☐ Both parents deceased due to old age
☐ Nocturia	☐ Father at age 89
☐ Duration 3 mos	☐ Mother at age 93
☐ Elevated PSA prompted biopsy	**Social Hx**
☐ No fever	☐ He is a retired attorney
☐ No chills	☐ Alcohol
☐ No fatigue	☐ 1-2 glasses of wine/week
☐ No polydipsia	☐ No recreational drugs
☐ No dysuria	☐ Except some marijuana in college
☐ No impotence	☐ No smoking
☐ No change in his bowel habits	☐ Sexually active with his wife only
☐ No change to appetite or weight.	☐ Has never been diagnosed with any sexually transmitted disease
☐ Eats a balanced diet	

Physical Examination

No physical exam

Patient Note

History

HPI: 68 y/o man with no significant past medical history presents to discuss results of his recent prostate biopsy. He reports developing increased urinary urgency, frequency, and hesitation over the past 3 mos, which was associated with weak urine stream and nocturia. He denies any change in urine color and dysuria, impotence, fatigue, fever, body aches and polydipsia. Additionally, there have been no changes in bowel habits, appetite or weight that were noted.

PMH/PSH: tonsillectomy at age 13

Meds: multivitamins

Allergies: NKDA

FHx: father and mother deceased due to old age, at age 89 and 93, respectively

SH: retired attorney, married, sexually active with wife. Social alcohol use, 1-2 drinks/week, no tobacco use, occasional marijuana use in college, eats a balanced diet

Physical Exam

There is no physical examination in this case.

Data Interpretation

DIAGNOSIS 1. ADENOCARCINOMA OF THE PROSTATE

History Findings	Physical Exam Findings
Urinary urgency, frequency and hesitancy	No physical exam
Weak urine stream	
Nocturia	
Elevated PSA	
Positive biopsy results	

Diagnostic Studies

Physical exam

Bone scan

CT scan of abd and pelvis

CASE 31: WEAKNESS

Doorway Information

Opening Scenario

Kristen Shore is a 24-year-old woman who comes to the office complaining of weakness for 2 months.

Vital Signs

T 37.2 C (98.9 F)

BP 115/77 mm Hg

Pulse 67/min

Respirations 16/min

Examinee Tasks

1. Obtain a focused history.

2. Perform a relevant physical exam. Do not perform rectal, pelvic, genitourinary, female breast, or corneal reflex exam.

3. Discuss your initial diagnostic impression and your workup plan with the patient.

4. After leaving the room, complete your patient note.

Communication and Interpersonal Skills Checklist

Fostering the Relationship	Gathering Information	Providing Information
☐ Knocked	☐ Elicited chief complaint	☐ Summarized significant information
☐ Introduced self	☐ Established timeline of patient's CC (chief complaint)	☐ Provided diagnostic impression
☐ Clarified role	☐ Used open-ended question	☐ Justified diagnosis with evidence from encounter
☐ Was properly groomed	☐ Used non-leading questions	☐ Assessed patient's need for additional information
☐ Made eye contact	☐ Used closed-ended questions	☐ Encouraged and answered questions
☐ Maintained appropriate distance	☐ Asked one question at a time	☐ Assessed patient's comprehension of probable illness
☐ Displayed confident manner	☐ Did not use medical jargon	
☐ Showed care and concern	☐ Appropriately used "continuers"	
☐ Was respectful and nonjudgmental	☐ Paraphrased	
☐ Established patient's preferred title	☐ Appropriately used transitions	
☐ Used proper draping	☐ Elicited additional concerns	
☐ Focused on patient	☐ Assessed impact on patient's life	
☐ Did not interrupt patient	☐ Checked for patient understanding	
☐ Maintained appropriate and responsive body language		

Making Decisions	Supporting Emotions
☐ Clearly stated next steps in management	☐ Actively listened and validated patient's expectations
☐ **Counseled** patient	☐ Showed empathy and used appropriate reassurances
☐ Agreed to **mutual plan** of action	☐ Inquired about patient's support system
	☐ Managed the **challenge** (here; patient is irritable)

History and Physical Examination Checklist

HPI

- ☐ Fatigue and weakness
  - ☐ Duration: 2 months
  - ☐ Progressive
- ☐ Blurry vision
- ☐ Double vision
  - ☐ Episodic
  - ☐ Worse when going up and down stairs
- ☐ Slurred speech
  - ☐ After a prolonged talk
- ☐ Jaw weakness
  - ☐ Difficulty chewing food
  - ☐ No difficulty swallowing
- ☐ Symptoms improve with rest
- ☐ Worse toward end of the day
- ☐ No headache
- ☐ No fever
- ☐ No chills
- ☐ No rash
- ☐ No joint pain
- ☐ No seizures
- ☐ No heat/cold intolerance
- ☐ No SOB
- ☐ Diarrhea
  - ☐ Episode prior to current symptoms
- ☐ No constipation
- ☐ No urinary changes
- ☐ No night sweats
- ☐ No weight change

PMH

- ☐ Recent infectious diarrhea
  - ☐ 2 months ago
- ☐ No hospitalization or surgery
- ☐ Meds: oral contraceptives
- ☐ NKDA
- ☐ LMP 2 weeks ago
- ☐ P0 G0

Family Hx

- ☐ Mother has hypothyroidism
- ☐ No other significant family history

Social Hx

- ☐ Mechanical engineering graduate student
- ☐ No recreational drugs
- ☐ No smoking
- ☐ No alcohol
- ☐ Single
  - ☐ Not sexually active

Physical Examination

- ☐ Washed hands prior to examination
- ☐ Examined oropharynx
- ☐ Assessed mental status
- ☐ Examined cranial nerves II–XII
  - ☐ Mild bilateral ptosis which is worsened by prolonged upward gaze
- ☐ Examined motor strength
- ☐ Examined sensation
- ☐ Examined DTRs
- ☐ Assessed gait
- ☐ Assessed cerebellar function
- ☐ Assessed plantar reflex
- ☐ Auscultated lungs

Patient Note

History

HPI: 24 yo woman presents c/o progressive weakness and fatigue x 2 months. The symptoms have become much worse over the past week. She also c/o blurry and double vision. It's worse when walking up and down the stairs and towards the end of the day. She has episodes of slurred speech and weakness with her jaw and chewing after eating or speaking for prolonged periods of time. Rest makes the symptoms better. She denies headache, fever, chills, rash, joint pains, seizure-like activity, heat or cold intolerance, palpitations, constipation, dysuria, or urinary frequency.

PMH: history of diarrhea 2 months ago

Medications: OCP

Allergies: NKDA

FHx: mother has hypothyroidism

SHx: does not drink, smoke, or use drugs; currently a graduate student; single and has never been pregnant, LMP 2 wks ago

Physical Examination

T 37.2 C (98.9 F); BP 115/77 mm Hg; pulse 67/min; respirations 16/min

GA: NAD

Oropharynx: no lesions

Lungs: CTA Bilaterally, no wheezes or crackles

Neuro: AAO x 3, PERRLA, mild bilateral ptosis which is worsened by prolonged upward gaze. CN II–XII intact, motor 5/5 UE/LE sensation intact to sharp/dull; plantar reflect WNL. DTRs 2+ and symmetric, no intention tremor or gait abnormalities, Romberg negative

Data Interpretation

Diagnosis 1. Myasthenia Gravis

History Findings	Physical Exam Findings
Progressive fatigue	Ptosis that worsens with prolonged upward gaze
Blurry vision/diplopia	Normal plantar reflex
Jaw weakness and weakness with chewing	
Slurred speech	
Female in third decade	
FH hypothyroidism	
Weakness increased w/ exertion and alleviated by rest	
Worsens as day progresses	

DIAGNOSIS 2. GUILLAIN-BARRE SYNDROME

History Findings	Physical Exam Findings
Progressive fatigue	Ptosis
Blurry vision/diplopia	Normal plantar reflex
Symptoms preceded by diarrheal illness	
Slurred speech	

DIAGNOSIS 3. BOTULISM

History Findings	Physical Exam Findings
Progressive fatigue	Ptosis
Blurry vision/diplopia	Normal plantar reflex
Jaw weakness and weakness with chewing	
Slurred speech	

Diagnostic Studies

Acetylcholine receptor antibodies

Muscle specific tyrosine kinase antibodies, anti-striated muscle antibodies (anti-SM)

Botulinum toxin blood test

FVC, negative inspiratory force (NIF)

Tensilon test

EMG, NCS

Chest x-ray

anti TK
anti SM abs

Appendix

Common Medical Abbreviations

Use abbreviations sparingly. For clarity, it is always better to spell out the acronym or abbreviation.

4Q	4 quadrants
yo or y/o	year old
m	male
f	female
b	black
w	white
L	left
R	right
hx	history
h/o	history of
c/o	complaining/complaints of
c	with
NL	normal limits
s	without
WNL	within normal limits
Ø	without or no
+	positive
–	negative

A&0x3	alert & oriented to person, place, and time
AA	Alcoholics Anonymous
AAA	abdominal aortic aneurysm
abd	abdomen

ABG	arterial blood gas
ACTH	adrenocorticotropic hormone
ADH	antidiuretic hormone
AFB	acid-fast bacilli
afib	atrial fibrillation
AIDS	acquired immune deficiency syndrome
Alb	albumin
Alk phos	alkaline phosphatase
ALS	amyotrophic lateral sclerosis
ant	anterior
A&P	auscultation and percussion
ARDS	acute respiratory distress syndrome
AV	arteriovenous
AP	anteroposterior
approx	approximately
ASA	aspirin

b/l	bilateral
BID	twice a day
BM	bowel movement
BP	blood pressure

BPH	benign prostatic hypertrophy
BUN	blood urea nitrogen
Bx	biopsy

Ca	calcium
CA	cancer
CABG	coronary artery bypass grafting
CAD	coronary artery disease
cath	catheterization
CBC	complete blood count
cc	chief complaint
CCU	cardiac care unit
CF	cystic fibrosis
Chemo	chemotherapy
CHF	congestive heart failure
chol	cholesterol
cig	cigarettes
Cl	chloride
CMV	cytomegalovirus
CN	cranial nerve
CNS	central nervous system
c/o	complains of
COPD	chronic obstructive pulmonary disease
CPK	creatine phosphokinase
CPR	cardiopulmonary resuscitation
Cr	creatinine
C&S, C/S	culture and sensitivity
CSF	cerebrospinal fluid
CT	computed tomography
CTA	clear to auscultation

CVA	cerebrovascular accident
CVP	central venous pressure
Cx	cervix
CXR	chest x-ray

D&C	dilatation and curettage
d/c	discontinue
DI	diabetes insipidus
DM	diabetes mellitus
DTR	deep tendon reflexes
DVT	deep vein thrombosis
dx	diagnosis

ECG/EKG	electrocardiogram
EEG	electroencephalogram
ED	emergency department
EGD	esophagogastroduodenoscopy
EMG	electromyogram
EMT	emergency medical technician
ENT	ears, nose, and throat
EOMI	extraocular muscles intact
ER	emergency room
ERCP	endoscopic retrograde cholangiopancreatography
ESR	erythrocyte sedimentation rate
EtOH	alcohol
ext	extremities

FBS	fasting blood sugar
Fe	iron

FSH	follicle stimulating hormone
FH	family history
FUO	fever of unknown origin
Fx	fracture

GA	general appearance
GERD	gastroesophageal reflux disorder
GI	gastrointestinal
Glu	glucose
GSW	gunshot wound
GTT	glucose tolerance test
GU	genitourinary

HA	headache
Hct	hematocrit
HEENT	head, eyes, ears, nose, and throat
Hgb	hemoglobin
HIV	human immunodeficiency virus
HRT	hormone replacement therapy
HPI	history of present illness
H. pylori	*Heliobacter pylori*
HR	heart rate
HSM	hepatosplenomegaly
HTN	hypertension

IBS	irritable bowel syndrome
ICU	intensive care unit
IDDM	insulin-dependent diabetes mellitus
IM	intramuscularly

INR	international ratio
IUD	intrauterine device
IV	intravenously

JVD	jugular venous distension
JVP	jugular venous pressure

K	potassium
KUB	kidney, ureter, and bladder

LAD	lymphadenopathy or left anterior descending
LDH	lactate dehydrogenase
LE	lower extremity
LH	luteinizing hormone
LLL	left lower lobe
LLQ	left lower quadrant
LMP	last menstrual period
loc	loss of consciousness
LP	lumbar puncture
LUL	left upper lobe
LUQ	left upper quadrant

M, R, G	murmurs, rubs, or gallops
meds	medications
mets	metastases
MI	myocardial infarction
MRI	magnetic resonance imaging
MS	multiple scleroris
MVA	motor vehicle accident
MVP	mitral valve prolapse

Na	sodium
NAD	no apparent distress
NC/AT	normocephalic atraumatic
neg	negative
neuro	neurologic
NIDDM	non–insulin-dependent diabetes mellitus
NKA	no known allergies
NKDA	no known drug allergy
NPH	normal pressure hydrocephalus
NSR	normal sinus rhythm
N/V	nausea and vomiting

PMI	point of maximum impulse
po	orally
pos	positive
PPD	packs per day
PPD	purified protein derivative
PRN	as needed
PSA	prostatic specific antigen
PT	prothrombin time
PTT	partial prothrombin time
PUD	peptic ulcer disease
PVD	peripheral vascular disease

occ	occasional
OCP	oral contraceptives
OD	right eye
OS	left eye
OTC	over-the-counter

r/o	rule out
RA	rheumatoid arthritis
RBC	red blood cells
RLL	right lower lobe
RLQ	right lower quadrant
RMG	rubs, murmurs, or gallops
ROM	range of motion
RR	respiratory rate
RRR	regular rate and rhythm
RUL	right upper lobe
RUQ	right upper quadrant
Rx	prescription

PA	posteroanterior
PCP	primary care provider
PCP	*pneumocystis carinii* pneumonia
PE	physical examination
PE	pulmonary embolus
PERRLA	pupils are equal, round, and reactive to light and accommodation
PET scan	positron emission tomography
PFTs	pulmonary function tests
PID	pelvic inflammatory disease

SH	social history
SLE	systemic lupus erythematosus
SLR	straight leg raising
sob	shortness of breath
SQ	subcutaneous

Staph	staphylococcus
STD	sexually transmitted disease
Strep	streptococcus

T	temperature
TB	tuberculosis
TIA	transient ischemic attack
TSH	thyroid stimulating hormone
TURP	transurethral prostatectomy
TVF	tactile vocal fremitus

U/A	urinalysis
UE	upper extremity
UGI	upper gastrointestinal
URI	upper respiratory tract infection
U/S	ultrasound
UTI	urinary tract infection

vag	vaginal
VCUG	voiding cystourethrogram
VDRL	Venereal Disease Research Laboratory
vs	vital signs

w/	with
WBC	white blood cells
wks	weeks
WNL	within normal limits
wt	weight